The Ultimate Vegetarian Soup Cookbook

Easy And Delicious Vegetarian Soups For Everyone

Adam Denton

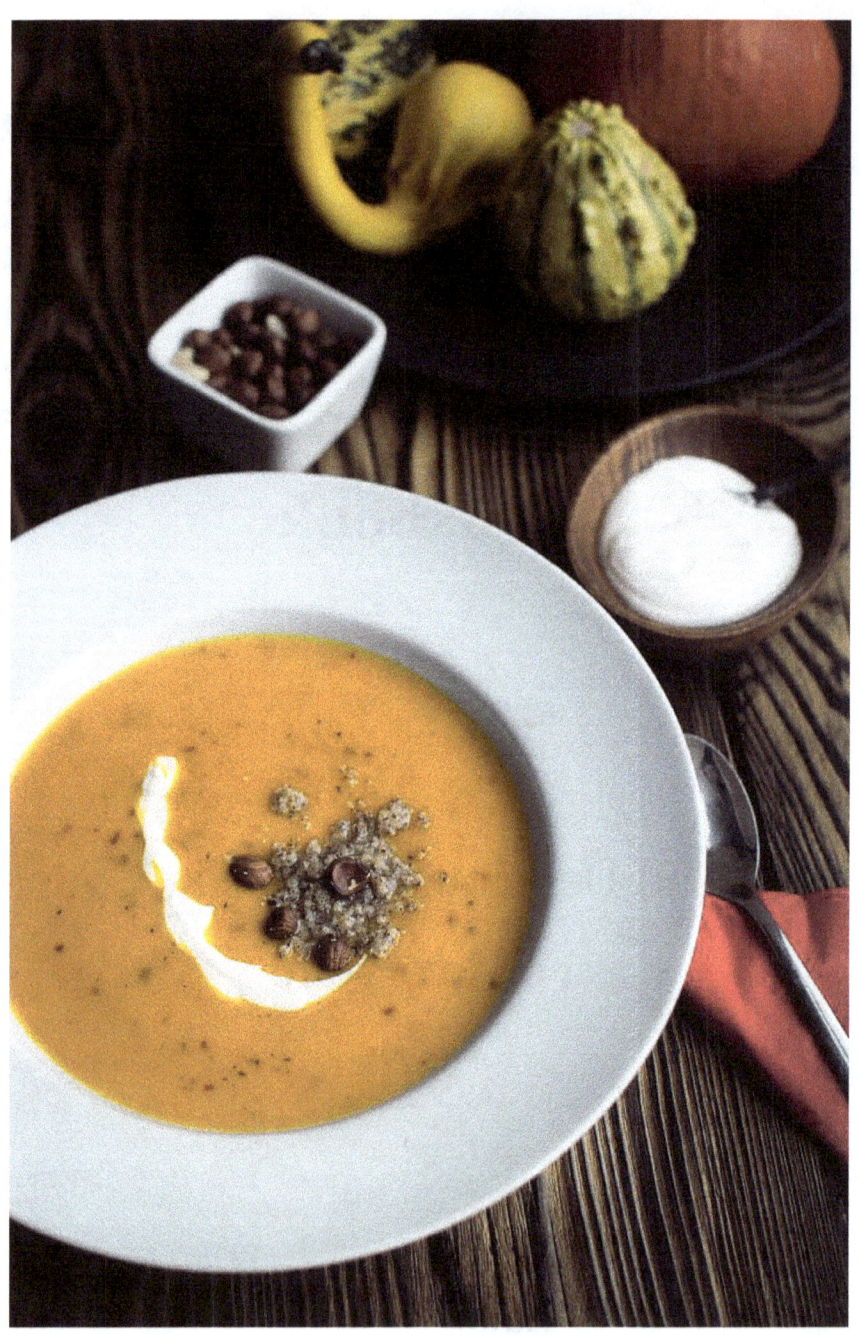

© **Copyright 2020 - All rights reserved.**

The content contained within this book may not be reproduced, duplicated or transmitted without direct written permission from the author or the publisher.

Under no circumstances will any blame or legal responsibility be held against the publisher, or author, for any damages, reparation, or monetary loss due to the information contained within this book. Either directly or indirectly.

Legal Notice:

This book is copyright protected. This book is only for personal use. You cannot amend, distribute, sell, use, quote or paraphrase any part, or the content within this book, without the consent of the author or publisher.

Disclaimer Notice:

Please note the information contained within this document is for educational and entertainment purposes only. All effort has been executed to present accurate, up to date, and reliable, complete information. No warranties of any kind are declared or implied. Readers acknowledge that the author is not engaging in the rendering of legal, financial, medical or professional advice. The content within this book has been derived from various sources. Please consult a licensed professional before attempting any techniques outlined in this book.

By reading this document, the reader agrees that under no circumstances is the author responsible for any losses, direct or indirect, which are incurred as a result of the use of information contained within this document, including, but not limited to, — errors, omissions, or inaccuracies.

Table of contents

Oriental Butternut Squash Soup 7

Squash and Ginger Soup (zucchini) 9

Buttery Butternut Squash and Lentil Soup 11

Creamy Almond and Turnip Soup 13

Buttery Carrot Soup 15

Italian Carrot Soup 17

Hungarian Carrot and Onion Soup 18

Spanish Vegan Chorizo and Carrot Soup 20

Vegan Chorizo and Sun-dried Tomato Soup 21

Sweet Potato and Lima Bean Soup 23

Italian Black Bean and Potato Soup 25

Borlotti Bean and Sun-dried Tomato Soup 27

Winter Squash Carrot and Parsnip Soup 29

Carrot Apple and Summer Squash Soup 31

Hubbard Squash Mushroom and Red Onion Soup 33

Summer Squash Carrot and Red Onion Soup 34

Garbanzo Bean Thai Curry Soup 36

Pinto Bean Jalapeno Soup 38

Lentil Tortilla Soup 40

Mexican Garbanzo Bean Soup 42

Watercress and Carrot Soup 44

Thai Turnip and Sweet Potato Soup 46

Summer Squash and Lemon Grass Soup 48

Summer Squash and Winter Soup 50

Creamy Parsnip and Peanut Soup Poblano Soup 51

Lentil and Butternut Squash Curry Soup 54

Thai Curried Butternut Squash Soup 56

Simple Carrot and Tarragon Soup 58

Thai Carrot Soup 60

Hungarian Carrot Soup 62

French Red Soup 63

Vidalia Onion and Parsnip Soup 65

Salad Tomato and Carrot Soup 67

Baby Potato and Garbanzo Bean Soup 69

French Baby Potato and Chick Pea Soup 71

Soybean Soup 73

Edamame Bean Soup 75

Peas and Kidney Bean Soup with Parsnips 77

Winter Squash and Turnip Soup 79

Winter Squash and Carrot Soup 81

Hubbard Squash and Parsnip Soup 83

Curried Winter Squash Curry 84

Garbanzo Bean Tortilla and Taco Soup 86

Lentils and Annatto Seed Tortilla Soup 88

Habanero Mung Bean Taco Soup 90

Borlotti Bean and Pepper Soup 92

Turnip and Chili Soup 94

Spicy Squash Soup 96

Jalapeno Butternut Squash Soup 98

Miso Summer Squash and Sweet Potato Soup 100

Middle Eastern Inspired Creamy Squash Soup 102

Habanero and Ancho Chili Sweet Potato Soup 105

Oriental Butternut Squash Soup

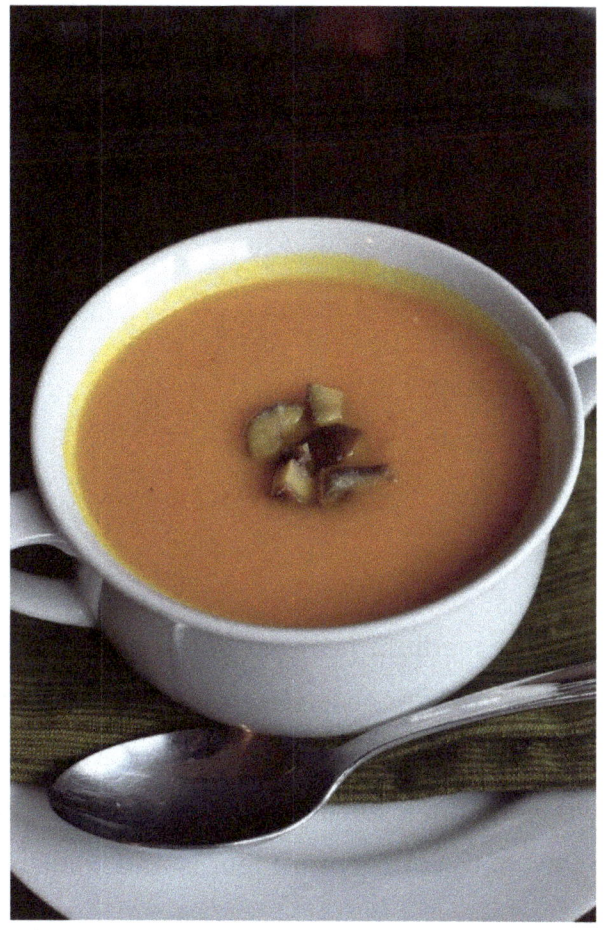

Ingredients

1 tablespoon sesame seed oil

1 small red onion, chopped

1 tablespoon minced fresh ginger root

4 cloves garlic, chopped

1 pinch Sichuan peppercorns

1 cup dry red lentils

1 cup butternut squash - peeled, seeded, and cubed

1/3 cup finely chopped fresh cilantro

2 cups water

1/2 (14 ounce) can almond milk

1 teaspoon red curry powder

¼ tsp. cayenne pepper

1 pinch ground nutmeg

salt and pepper to taste

Directions:

Heat the pot over medium heat Sauté the onion, ginger, garlic, until onion is tender. Add the lentils, squash, and cilantro into the pot. Add the water, almond milk, and tomato paste. Add the curry powder, cayenne pepper, nutmeg, salt, and pepper. Boil, reduce the heat to low, and simmer until lentils and squash are tender for 25 min.

Squash and Ginger Soup (zucchini)

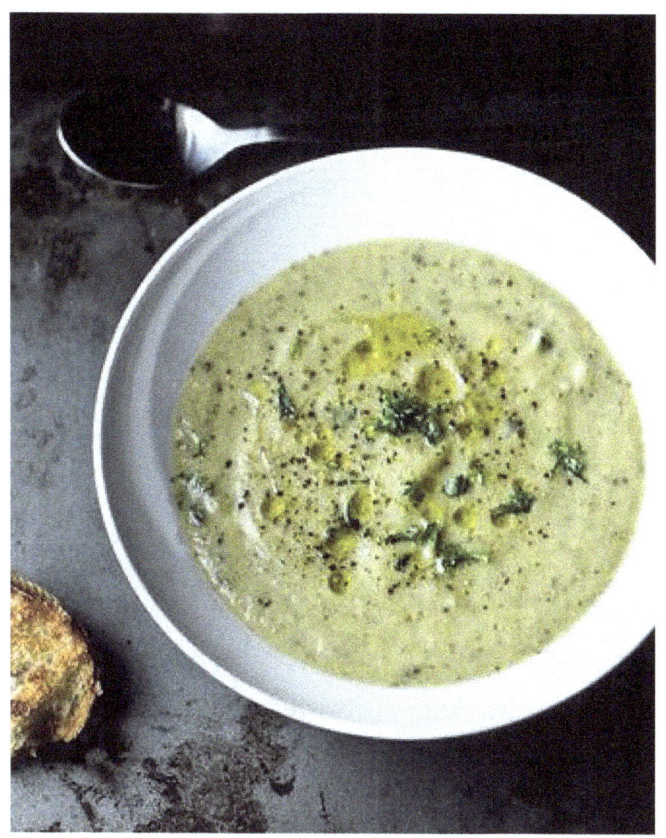

Ingredients

1 tablespoon extra virgin olive oil

1 small red onion, chopped

1 tablespoon minced fresh ginger root

5 cloves garlic, chopped

1 pinch fenugreek seeds

1 cup dry red lentils

1 cup Zucchini - peeled, seeded, and cubed

1/3 cup finely chopped fresh cilantro

2 cups water

1/2 (14 ounce) can milk

2 tablespoons tomato paste

1 teaspoon red curry powder

¼ tsp. cayenne pepper

1 pinch ground nutmeg

salt and pepper to taste

Directions:

Heat the pot over medium heat Sauté the onion, ginger, garlic, and fenugreek until onion is tender. Add the lentils, zucchini, and cilantro into the pot. Add the water, coconut milk, and tomato paste. Add the curry powder, cayenne pepper, nutmeg, salt, and pepper. Boil, reduce the heat to low, and simmer until lentils and zucchini are tender for 25 min.

Buttery Butternut Squash and Lentil Soup

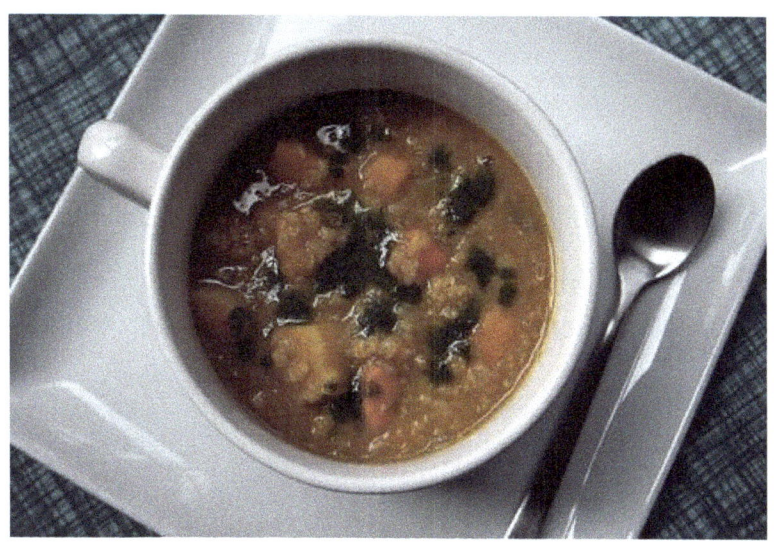

Ingredients

1 tablespoon butter

1 small red onion, chopped

4 cloves garlic, chopped

1 cup dry red lentils

1 cup butternut squash - peeled, seeded, and cubed

2 cups vegetable broth

1/2 (14 ounce) can milk

1 teaspoon thyme

¼ tsp. marjoram

1 pinch ground nutmeg

salt and pepper to taste

Directions:

Heat the pot over medium heat and melt the butter Sauté the onion, & garlic until onion is tender. Add the lentils & squash into the pot. Add the broth and almond milk. Add the thyme, marjoram, nutmeg, salt, and pepper. Boil, reduce the heat to low, and simmer until lentils and squash are tender for 25 min.

Creamy Almond and Turnip Soup

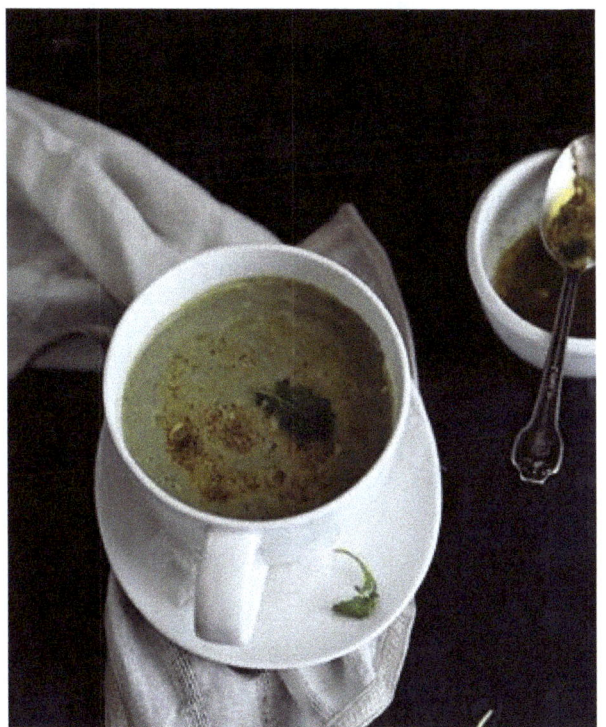

Ingredients

3 tablespoons salted butter

1 small red onion, minced

1 small turnip, peeled and thinly sliced

1 celery rib, thinly sliced 5 cloves garlic, minced

1 cup vegetable broth

1 cup almond milk

2 tbsp. white wine vinegar

Directions:

Melt butter over medium-high heat. Sauté onions until tender for about 5 minutes. Add turnip, celery, and garlic, and cook for another 5 minutes, or until carrots become tender. Add vegetable broth, almond milk and wine vinegar. Boil and reduce to a simmer, and cook for 15 minutes longer.

Buttery Carrot Soup

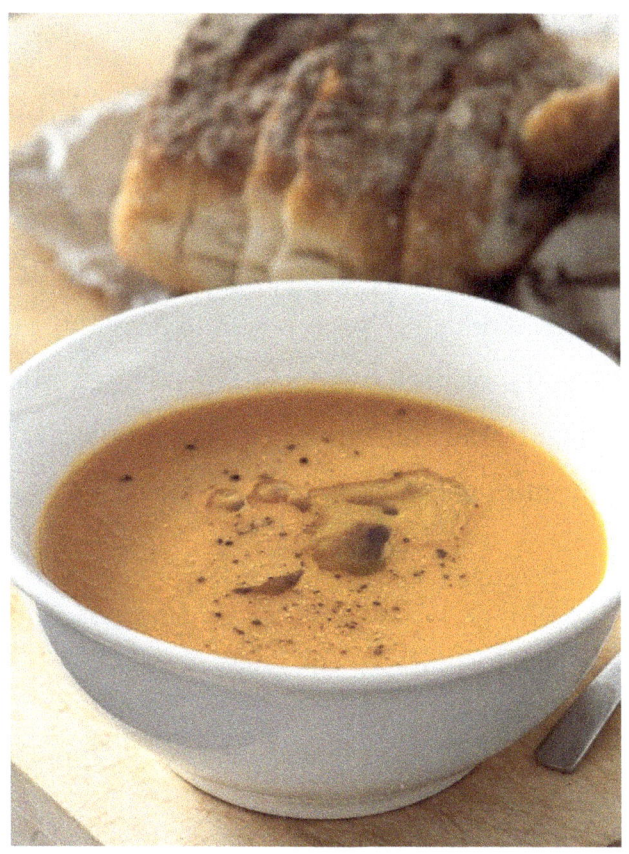

Ingredients

3 tablespoons butter

1 small yellow onion, minced

1 small parsnips, peeled and thinly sliced

1 celery rib, thinly sliced

1/2 teaspoon herbs de Provence

2 cups vegetable broth

2 tbsp. white wine vinegar

¼ cup heavy cream

Directions:

Heat oil over medium-high heat. Sauté onions until tender for about 5 minutes. Add parsnips, celery, and tarragon, and cook for another 5 minutes, or until carrots become tender. Add vegetable broth, cream and wine vinegar. Boil and reduce to a simmer, and cook for 15 minutes longer.

Italian Carrot Soup

Ingredients

3 tablespoons extra virgin olive oil

1 small red onion, minced

1 small carrot, peeled and thinly sliced

1 celery rib, thinly sliced

1 tbsp. minced garlic

1/2 teaspoon Italian seasoning

2 cups vegetable broth

¼ cup pesto

2 tbsp. white wine vinegar

Directions:

Heat oil over medium-high heat. Sauté onions until tender for about 5 minutes. Add carrots, celery, garlic and Italian seasoning, and cook for another 5 minutes, or until carrots become tender. Add vegetable broth and wine vinegar. Boil and reduce to a simmer, add the pesto and cook for 15 minutes longer.

Hungarian Carrot and Onion Soup

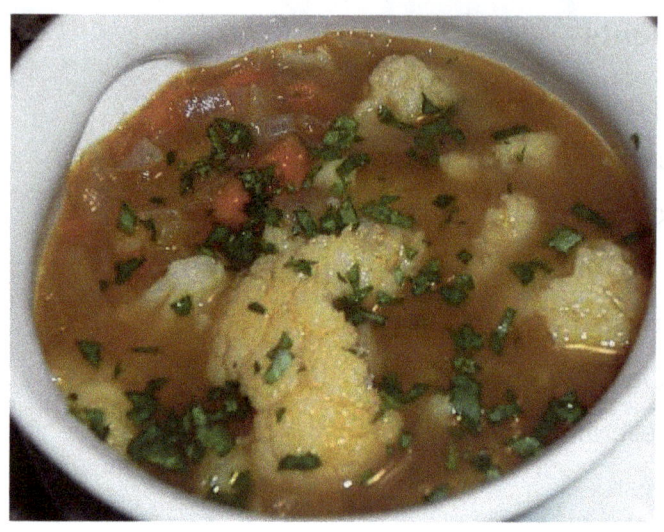

Ingredients

3 tablespoons salted butter

1 large red onion, minced

1 small carrot, peeled and thinly sliced

1 potato, thinly sliced

1/2 teaspoon Hungarian paprika

1 cup vegetable broth

1 cup almond milk

2 tbsp. white wine vinegar

Directions:

Heat melted butter over medium-high heat. Sauté onions until tender for about 5 minutes. Add carrot, potato, and paprika, and cook for another 5 minutes, or until carrot become tender. Add vegetable broth and almond milk. Boil and reduce to a simmer, and cook for 15 minutes longer.

Spanish Vegan Chorizo and Carrot Soup

Ingredients

3 tablespoons extra virgin olive oil

1 small Vidalia onion, minced

1 small carrot, peeled and thinly sliced 1 vegan chorizo, coarsely chopped (Soyrizo brand)

1 tbsp. dried Spanish paprika 1 tsp. thyme

2 cups vegetable broth

2 tbsp. white wine vinegar Parsley for garnishing

Directions:

Heat oil over medium-high heat. Sauté onions until tender for about 5 minutes. Add carrots, vegan chorizo, and tarragon, and cook for another 5 minutes, or until carrots become tender. Add vegetable broth, paprika, thyme and wine vinegar. Boil and reduce to a simmer, and cook for 15 minutes longer. Garnish with parsley Sun-dried

Vegan Chorizo and Sun-dried Tomato Soup

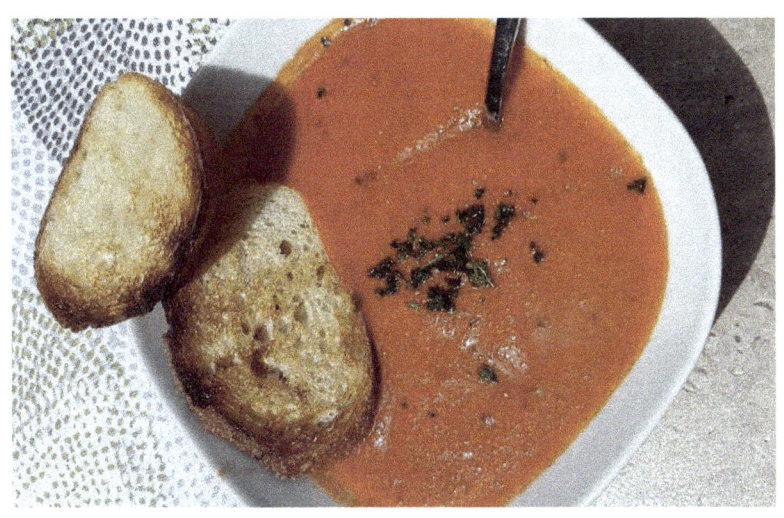

Ingredients

1 pound lentils, sorted and rinsed

1 1/2 quarts vegetable stock

½ quart water

1 medium red onion, diced

6 cloves of garlic, peeled and smashed 1 vegan chorizo (brand: Soyrizo), coarsely chopped

2 tsp sea salt

1/4 tsp pepper

2 medium potatoes, diced

1 pound frozen, sliced carrots

1 cup chopped sun-dried tomatoes* 1 tsp saffron

2 tsp. Spanish Paprika

3-4 tbsp fresh, minced parsley

Directions:

Add the lentils, veggie stock and water, onion, garlic, salt and pepper in a pot and cook over low-medium heat. Simmer for 3-4 hours. When the lentils become soft, add the potato and simmer until the potatoes become tender. Add the carrots, tomatoes, vegan chorizo, paprika and saffron and cook until heated through. Add the parsley. Season with more salt and pepper.

Sweet Potato and Lima Bean Soup

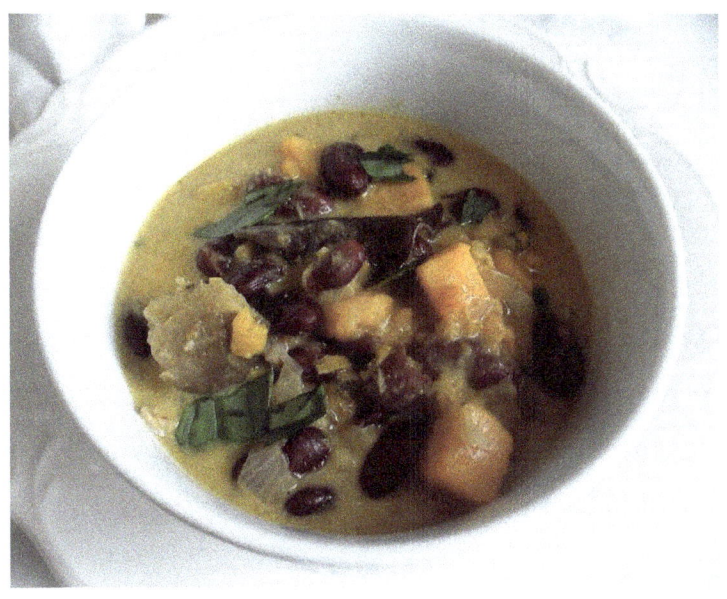

Ingredients

1 pound dry lima beans, sorted and rinsed

1 1/2 quarts vegetable broth

½ quart water

1 medium onion, diced

6 cloves of garlic, peeled and smashed

2 tsp sea salt

1/4 tsp pepper

2 medium sweet potatoes, diced

1 pound frozen, sliced carrots 1-

2 tsp balsamic vinegar

3-4 tbsp fresh, minced parsley

Directions:

Add the beans, vegetable broth and water, onion, garlic, salt and pepper in a pot and cook over low-medium heat. Simmer for 3-4 hours. When the beans become soft, add the potato and simmer until the potatoes become tender. Add the carrots, tomatoes and balsamic vinegar and cook until heated through. Add the parsley. Season with more salt and pepper.

Italian Black Bean and Potato Soup

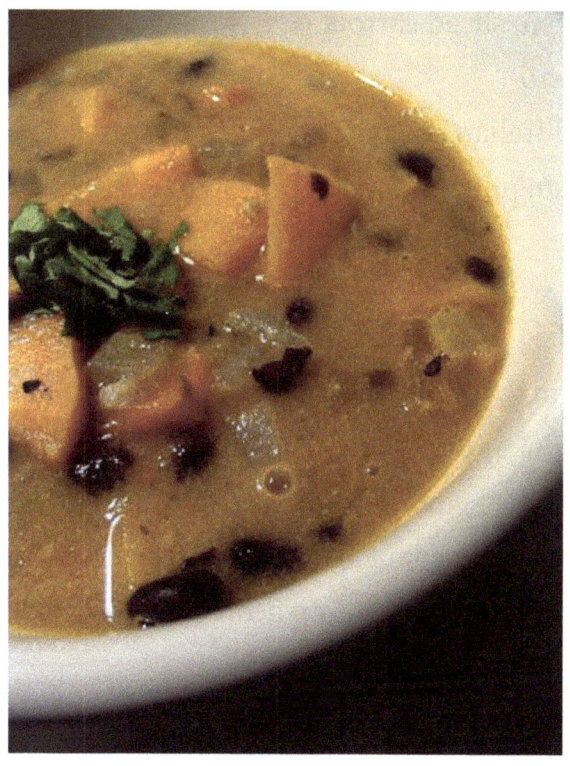

Ingredients

1 pound black beans, sorted and rinsed

1 1/2 quarts vegetable broth

½ quart water

1 medium red onion, diced

8 cloves of garlic, peeled and smashed

2 tsp sea salt

1/4 tsp pepper

2 medium potatoes, diced

1 pound frozen, sliced carrots

1 cup red pesto

1-2 tsp dried Italian seasoning

3-4 tbsp fresh, minced parsley

Directions:

Add the beans, veggie stock and water, onion, garlic, salt and pepper in a pot and cook over low-medium heat. Simmer for 3-4 hours. When the beans become soft, add the potato and simmer until the potatoes become tender. Add the carrots, red pesto, and Italian seasoning and cook until heated through. Add the parsley. Season with more salt and pepper.

Borlotti Bean and Sun-dried Tomato Soup

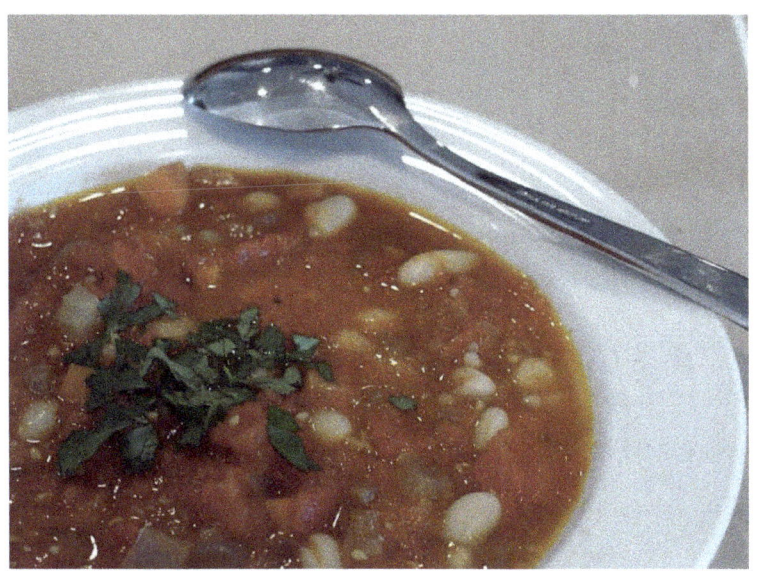

Ingredients

1 pound borlotti beans, sorted and rinsed

1 1/2 quarts vegetable stock

½ quart water

1 medium onion, diced

9 cloves of garlic, peeled and smashed

2 tsp sea salt

1/4 tsp pepper

2 medium potatoes, diced

1 pound frozen, sliced carrots

1 cup chopped sun-dried tomatoes*

1-2 tsp lime juice

3-4 tbsp fresh, minced parsley

Directions:

Add the beans, veggie stock and water, onion, garlic, salt and pepper in a pot and cook over low-medium heat. Simmer for 3-4 hours. When the beans become soft, add the potato and simmer until the potatoes become tender. Add the carrots, tomatoes and lime juice and cook until heated through. Add the parsley. Season with more salt and pepper.

Winter Squash Carrot and Parsnip Soup

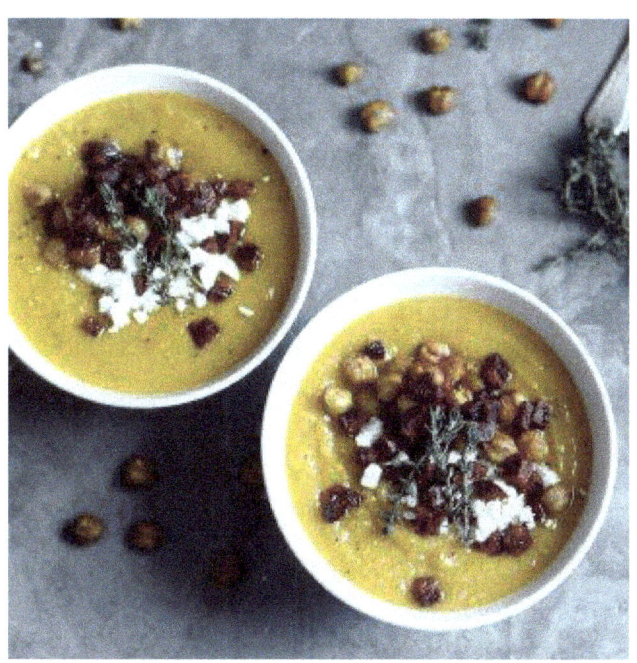

Ingredients

1 medium wintersquash squash (1 lb of peeled and cubed butternut squash)

1 medium red onion, diced

1/2 lb carrots, peeled and cut into chunks

1 parsnip, peeled and sliced

2 cups vegetable stock

1 tsp salt

1 tsp pepper

2 (13.5 oz) cans almond milk

salt and pepper to taste

Directions:

Combine the squash, red onion, parsnips, carrots, & stock in slow cooker. Cook for about 6 hours on low or until veggies are soft. Transfer the Ingredients of the slow cooker to a blender Blend until smooth. Pour back into the slow cooker and season with salt, pepper & sage Add the almond milk. Stir. Taste and season with more salt and pepper to taste.

Carrot Apple and Summer Squash Soup

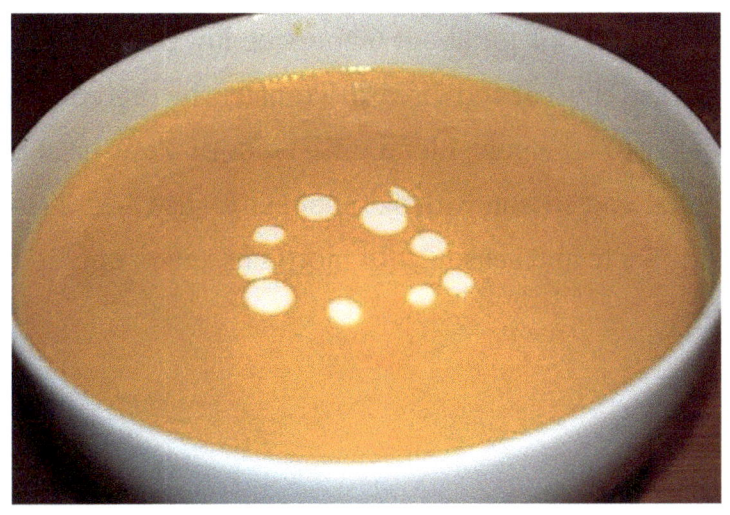

Ingredients

1 medium summer squash

1 medium red onion, diced

1/2 lb carrots, peeled and cut into chunks

1 Fuji apple, peeled and sliced

3 cups vegetable stock

1 bay leaf

1 tsp salt

1 tsp pepper

1/4 tsp dried ground sage

1 (13.5 oz) can almond milk

salt and pepper to taste

Directions:

Combine the squash, red onion, carrots, apple, stock and bay leaf in slow cooker. Cook for about 6 hours on low or until veggies are soft. Take the bay leaf and discard. Transfer the Ingredients of the slow cooker to a blender Blend until smooth. Pour back into the slow cooker and season with salt, pepper & sage Add the almond milk. Stir. Taste and season with more salt and pepper to taste.

Hubbard Squash Mushroom and Red Onion Soup

Ingredients

1 lb. Hubbard squash

1 medium red onion, diced

1/2 lb carrots, peeled and cut into chunks

1 can (14 oz.) mushrooms, sliced

3 cups vegetable stock

1 bay leaf

1 tsp salt

1 tsp pepper

2 sprigs rosemary

salt and pepper to taste

Directions:

Combine the squash, red onion, carrots, mushrooms, stock and rosemary in slow cooker. Cook for about 6 hours on low or until veggies are soft. Take the bay leaf and discard. Transfer the Ingredients of the slow cooker to a blender Blend until smooth. Pour back into the slow cooker and season with salt & pepper Taste and season with more salt and pepper to taste.

Summer Squash Carrot and Red Onion Soup

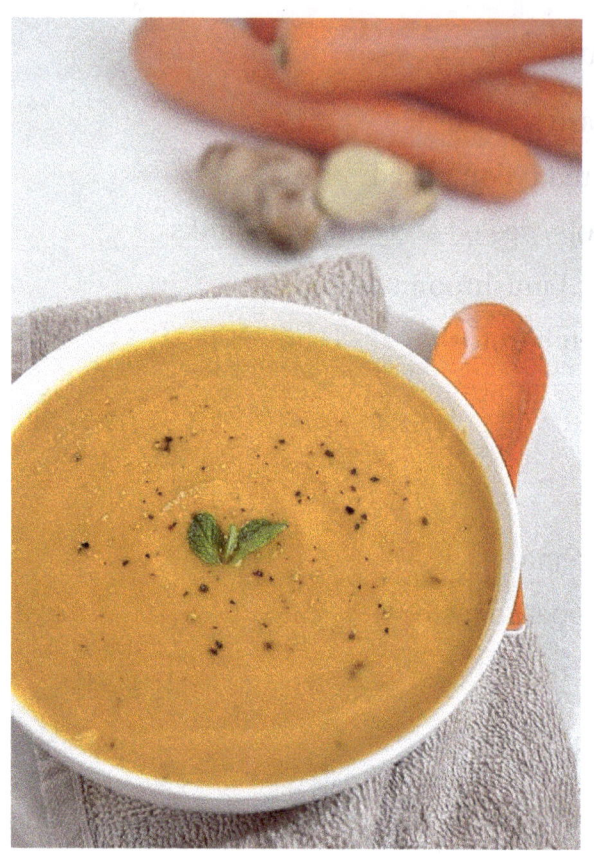

Ingredients

1 medium summer squash (1 lb of peeled and cubed butternut squash)

1 medium red onion, diced

1/2 lb carrots, peeled and cut into chunks

3 cups vegetable stock

1 tsp salt

1 tsp pepper

1/4 tsp cumin

½ (6.5 oz) can tomatoes

salt and pepper to taste

Directions:

Combine the squash, red onion, carrots, & stock in slow cooker. Cook for about 6 hours on low or until veggies are soft. Transfer the Ingredients of the slow cooker to a blender Blend until smooth. Pour back into the slow cooker and season with salt, pepper & cumin Add the tomatoes. Stir. Taste and season with more salt and pepper to taste.

Garbanzo Bean Thai Curry Soup

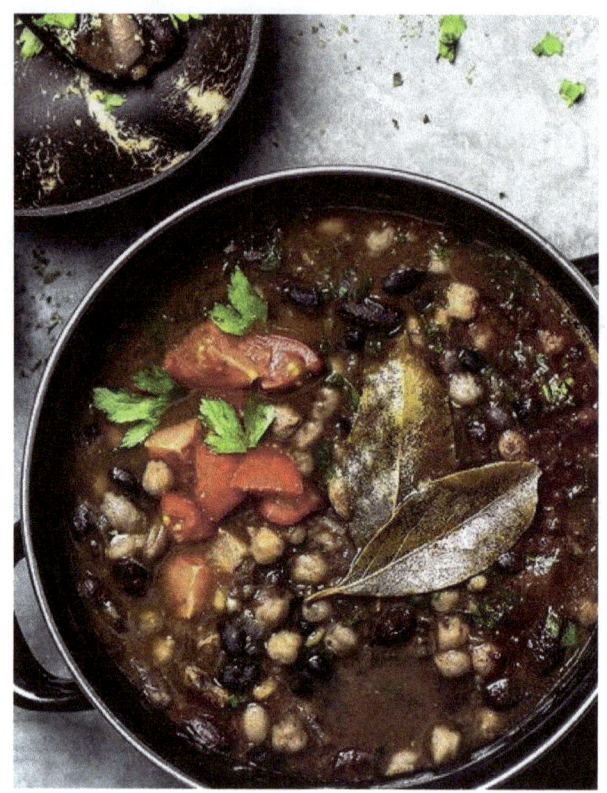

Ingredients

1 teaspoon olive oil

1/2 cup chopped red onions

4 cloves garlic, minced

2 cups vegetable broth

1 tsp. curry powder

1 14-ounce can garbanzo beans

1/2 teaspoon sea salt

1 cup coconut milk

1/2 cup loosely-packed coriander

Directions:

Heat the olive oil on medium. Add the red onions and garlic to the pan and stir until softened, 3 to 5 minutes. Pour in broth, curry powder, bell peppers, black beans, coriander coconut milk and salt. Boil over high heat. Reduce heat to low and simmer until heated through for about 5 minutes.

Pinto Bean Jalapeno Soup

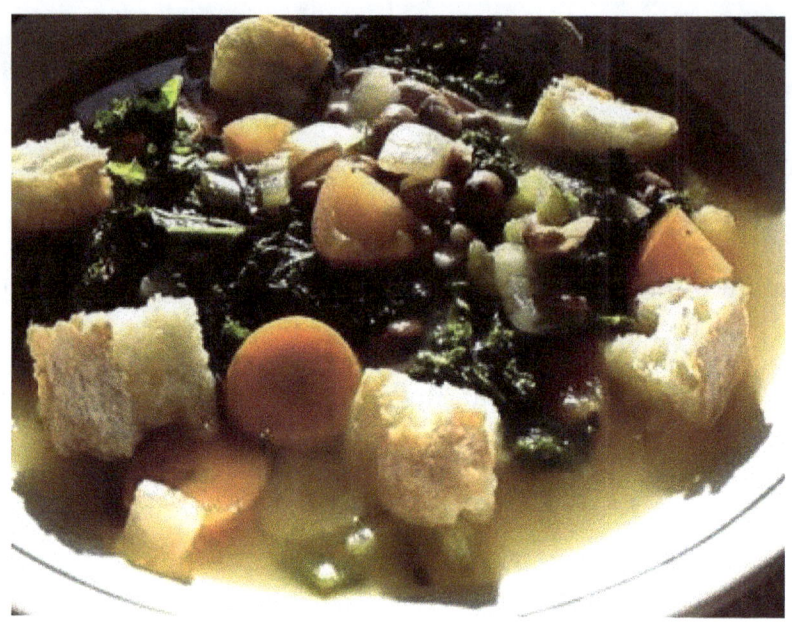

Ingredients:

1 teaspoon extra virgin olive oil

1/2 cup chopped yellow onions

4 cloves garlic, minced

2 cups vegetable broth

1 cup salsa

1 14-ounce can pinto beans

¼ cup jalapeno peppers, chopped

1/2 teaspoon sea salt

1 cup corn

1 tsp. chili powder

Directions:

Heat the olive oil on medium. Add the yellow onions and garlic to the pan and stir until softened, 3 to 5 minutes. Pour in broth, salsa, jalapeno peppers, black beans, and salt. Boil over high heat. Reduce heat to low and simmer until heated through for about 5 minutes. Top with the corn & chili powder.

Lentil Tortilla Soup

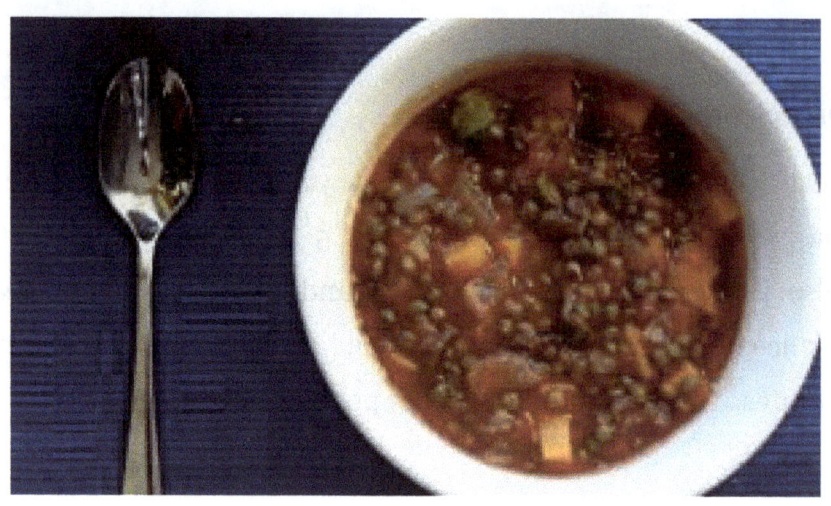

Ingredients:

1 teaspoon extra virgin olive oil

1/2 cup chopped red onions

4 cloves garlic, minced

2 cups vegetable broth

1 cup salsa

1 tsp. Louisiana style hot sauce

1 14-ounce can lentils

1 jalapeno , chopped

1/2 teaspoon sea salt 1 avocado, chopped

1 tsp. cumin

½ tsp, coriander

Optional:

1/2 cup crumbled corn tortilla chips

Chop onions and garlic.

Chop red bell pepper.

Directions:

Heat the olive oil on medium. Add the red onions and garlic to the pan and stir until softened, 3 to 5 minutes. Pour in broth, salsa, hot sauce, jalapeno peppers, black beans, cumin, coriander and salt. Boil over high heat. Reduce heat to low and simmer until heated through for about 5 minutes. Top with half of the avocado, cilantro, and tortilla chips.

Mexican Garbanzo Bean Soup

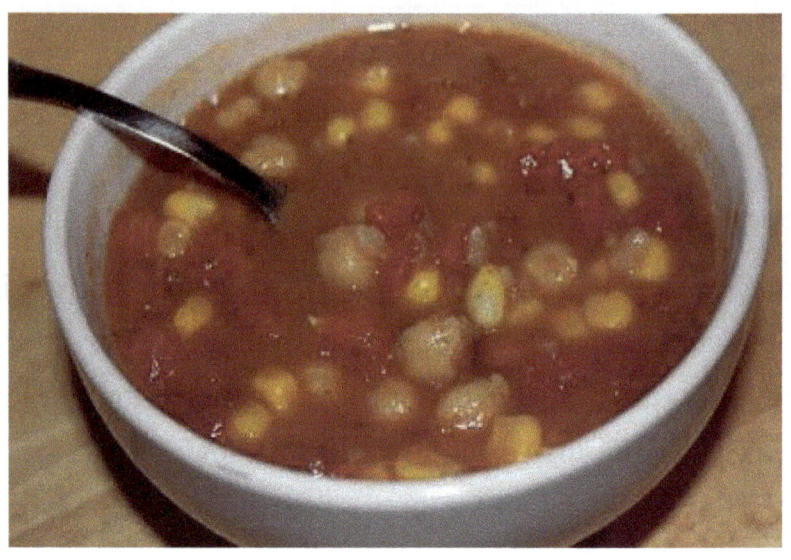

Ingredients:

1 teaspoon extra virgin olive oil

1/2 cup chopped red onions

4 cloves garlic, minced

2 cups vegetable broth

1 tsp. cumin

1 14-ounce can garbanzo beans

1 green bell pepper, chopped

1/2 teaspoon sea salt

1 tbsp. lime juice

1/2 cup loosely-packed cilantro

1 cup vegan chorizo, coarsely chopped

Directions:

Heat the olive oil on medium. Add the red onions and garlic to the pan and stir until softened, 3 to 5 minutes. Pour in broth, salsa, cumin, vegan chorizo, bell peppers, black beans, lime juice, and salt. Boil over high heat. Reduce heat to low and simmer until heated through for about 5 minutes.

Watercress and Carrot Soup

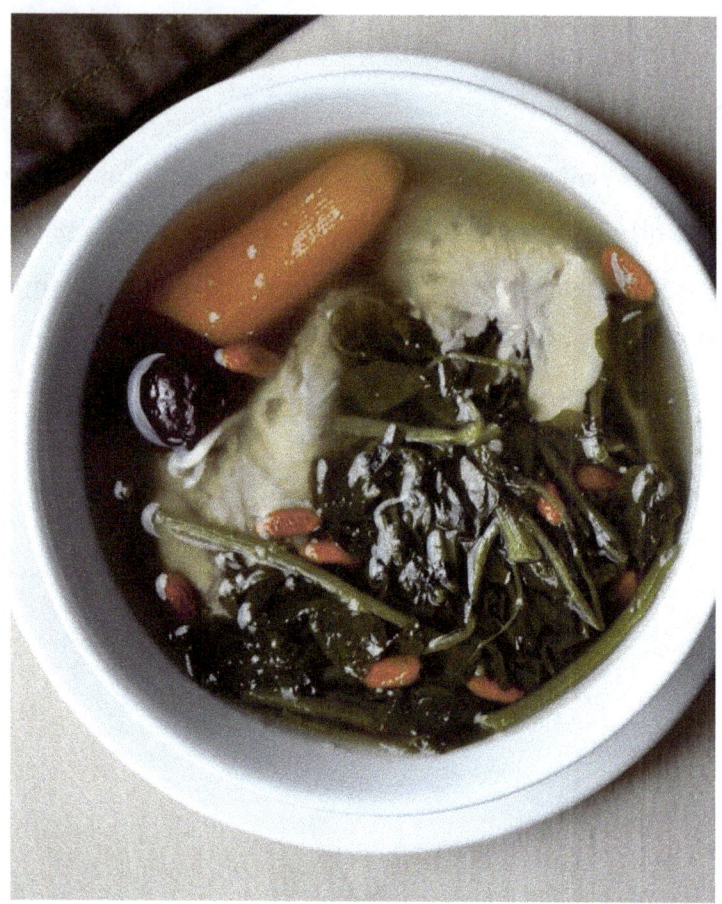

Ingredients

1 tablespoon sesame oil

3 teaspoons crushed garlic

1 tablespoon chopped fresh cilantro

2 teaspoons chili garlic sauce

1 red onion, chopped

3 large carrots, peeled and sliced

1 bunch watercress, coarsely chopped

5 cups vegetable stock

Directions:

Heat oil in a pot over medium heat. Cook garlic, cilantro and chili garlic sauce. Cook onions until tender. Add the carrots and watercress. Cook for 5 minutes and pour in vegetable stock. Simmer for 40 minutes, or until spinach and carrots become soft. Blend until smooth.

Thai Turnip and Sweet Potato Soup

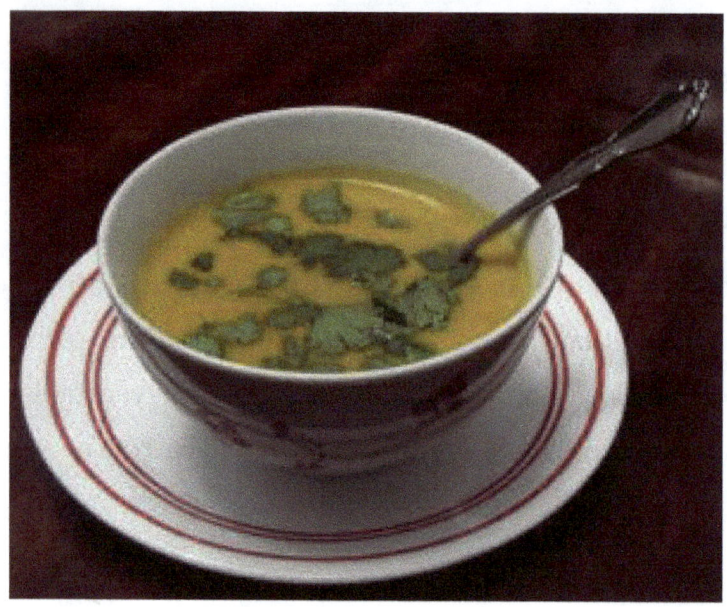

Ingredients

1 tablespoon sesame seed oil

3 teaspoons crushed garlic

1 tablespoon chopped fresh cilantro

1 teaspoon Thai bird chilies, minced

2 tbsp. tamarind paste

1 tsp. Thai chili paste

1 red onion, chopped

3 large turnips, peeled and sliced

1 large sweet potato, peeled and chopped

5 cups vegetable broth

Directions:

Heat oil in a pot over medium heat. Cook garlic, cilantro, Thai chilies, tamarind paste, and Thai chili paste. Cook onions until tender. Add the turnips and potato. Cook for 5 minutes and pour in vegetable stock. Simmer for 40 minutes, or until potatoes and turnips become soft. Blend until smooth.

Summer Squash and Lemon Grass Soup

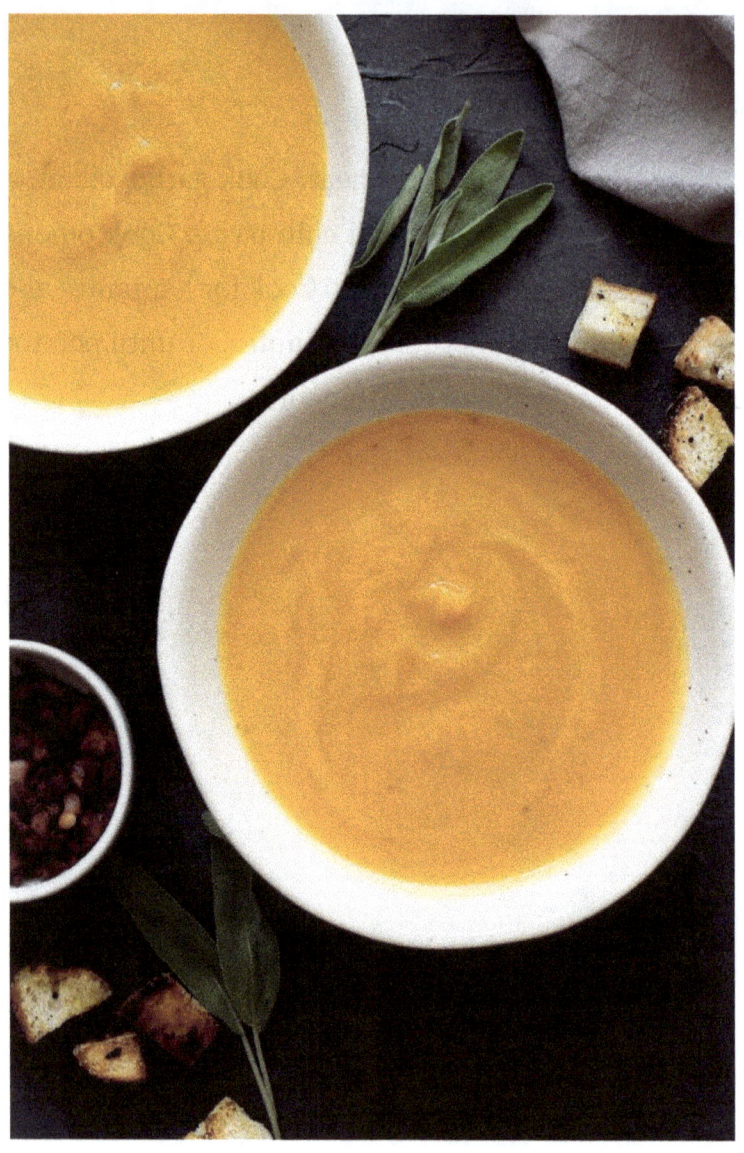

Ingredients

1 tablespoon extra-virgin olive oil

3 teaspoons crushed garlic

1 tablespoon chopped fresh cilantro

2 to 3 stalks lemon grass

1 tsp. ginger, finely minced

1 red onion, chopped

3 large summer squash, peeled and sliced

1 large potato, peeled and chopped

5 cups vegetable stock

Directions:

Heat oil in a pot over medium heat. Cook garlic, cilantro, lemon grass & ginger. Cook onions until tender. Add the squash and potato. Cook for 5 minutes and pour in vegetable stock. Simmer for 40 minutes, or until potatoes and squash become soft. Blend until smooth.

Summer Squash and Winter Soup

Ingredients

1 tablespoon sesame seed oil

7 teaspoons crushed garlic

1 tablespoon chopped fresh cilantro

1 teaspoon Chinese five spice powder

1 teaspoon chili garlic paste

1 red onion, chopped

3 large pcs. of summer squash, peeled and sliced

1 large winter squash, peeled and chopped

5 cups vegetable broth

Directions:

Heat oil in a pot over medium heat. Cook garlic, cilantro and chili paste. Cook onions until tender. Add the squash. Cook for 5 minutes and pour in vegetable stock. Simmer for 40 minutes, or until squash become soft. Blend until smooth.

Creamy Parsnip and Peanut Soup Poblano Soup

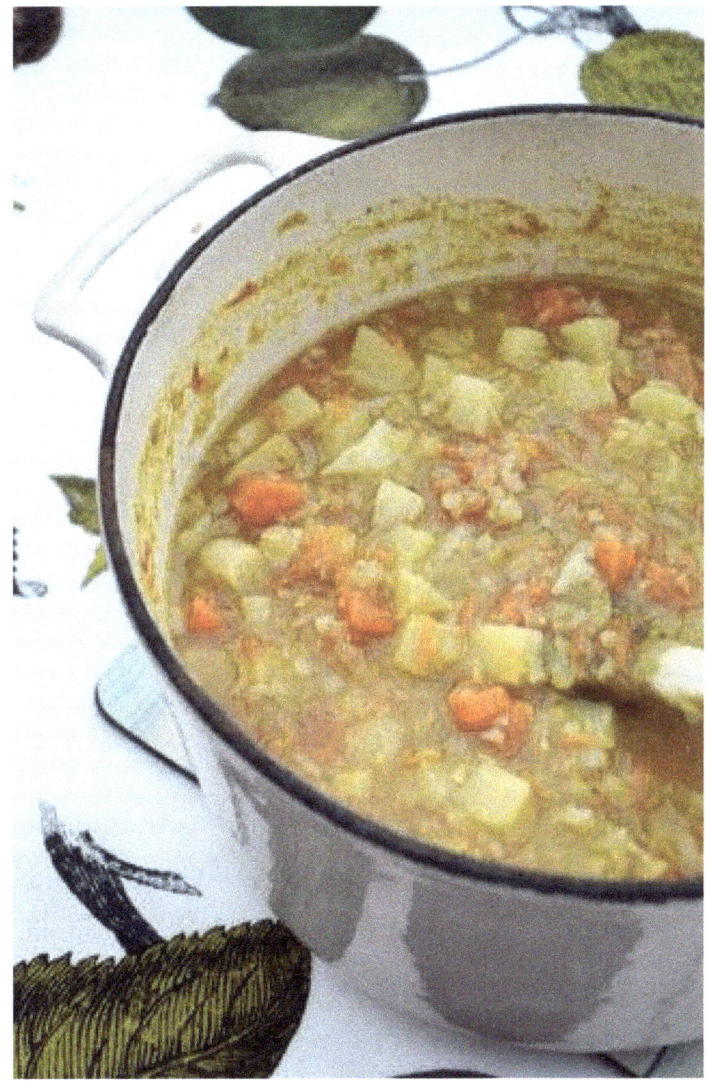

Ingredients:

4 tablespoons salted butter

1 small red onion, coarsely chopped

1 large leek, white part only, sliced

1 green bell pepper, coarsely chopped

5 pcs. Thai chilies, sliced

5 Thai basil leaves

2 tbsp. tamarind paste

8 cloves garlic, diced

1 large parsnip, cubed (you can use two if you like your soup thick)

4 cups vegetable broth

1 cup peanuts

1-1/4 coconut milk

Sea salt

Black pepper

Directions:

Optional garnish: Sliced jalapeno pepper Soak peanuts in almond milk for an hour. Melt non-dairy butter in a pan. Add the red onion, leek, chilies, Thai basil, tamarind paste, bell pepper, garlic, and potato. Cook on low heat and stir until the onion is translucent, 6 1/2 minutes. Add the broth into the pan. Simmer until the parsnip are fork tender for about 25 minutes. Take it off the heat. Process the mixture in a blender until smooth. Return the soup to the pan. In the blender, blend peanuts with coconut milk until smooth Add to the soup mixture. Heat the soup on medium heat for a few more minutes. Garnish with slices of jalapeno.

Lentil and Butternut Squash Curry Soup

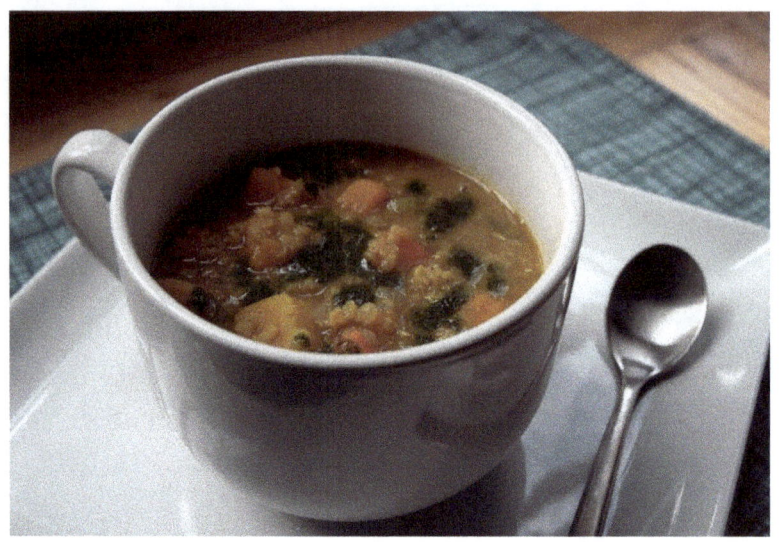

Ingredients

1 tablespoon sesame seed oil

1 small red onion, chopped

1 tablespoon minced fresh ginger root

3 cloves garlic, chopped

1 pinch fenugreek seeds

1 cup dry red lentils

1 cup butternut squash - peeled, seeded, and cubed

1/3 cup finely chopped fresh cilantro

2 cups water

1/2 (14 ounce) can almond milk

2 tablespoons tomato paste

1 teaspoon red curry powder

1/4 cayenne pepper

1 pinch ground nutmeg

salt and pepper to taste

Directions:

Heat the oil in a pot over medium heat Sauté the onion, garlic, and fenugreek until onion becomes tender. Add the lentils, squash, and cilantro into the pot. Add the water, almond milk, and tomato paste. Season with curry powder, cayenne pepper, nutmeg, salt, and pepper. Boil and reduce heat to low Simmer until lentils and squash are tender. For about 30 min.

Thai Curried Butternut Squash Soup

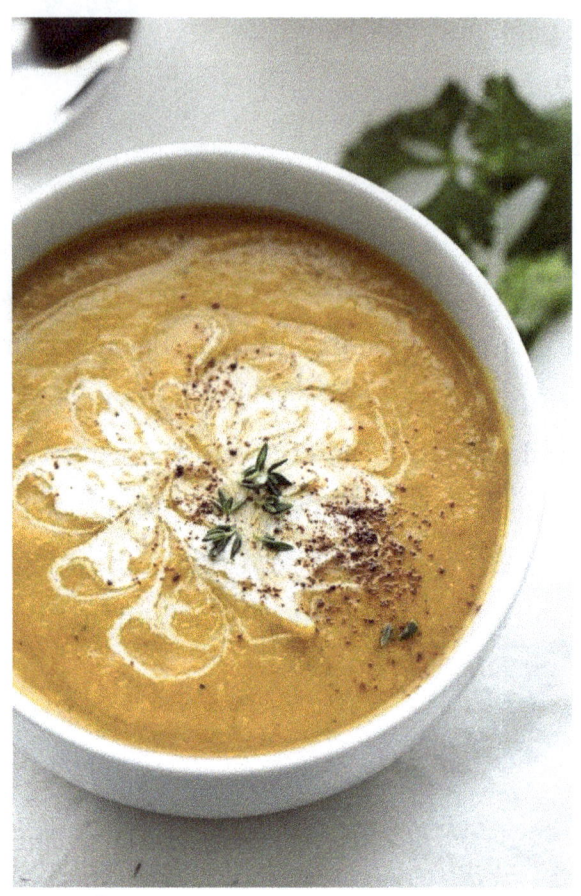

Ingredients

1 tablespoon sesame seed oil

1 small red onion, chopped

1 tablespoon minced fresh ginger root

3 cloves garlic, chopped

1 cup peanuts

1 cup butternut squash - peeled, seeded, and cubed

1/3 cup finely chopped fresh cilantro

2 cups water

1/2 (14 ounce) can coconut milk

1 teaspoon red curry powder

1tsp. Thai bird chilies

1 pinch ground nutmeg

salt and pepper to taste

Directions:

Heat the oil in a pot over medium heat Sauté the onion, ginger, and garlic until onion becomes tender. Add the peanuts, squash, and cilantro into the pot. Add the water & coconut milk. Season with curry powder, Thai bird chilies, nutmeg, salt, and pepper. Boil and reduce heat to low Simmer until peanuts and squash are tender. For about 30 min.

Simple Carrot and Tarragon Soup

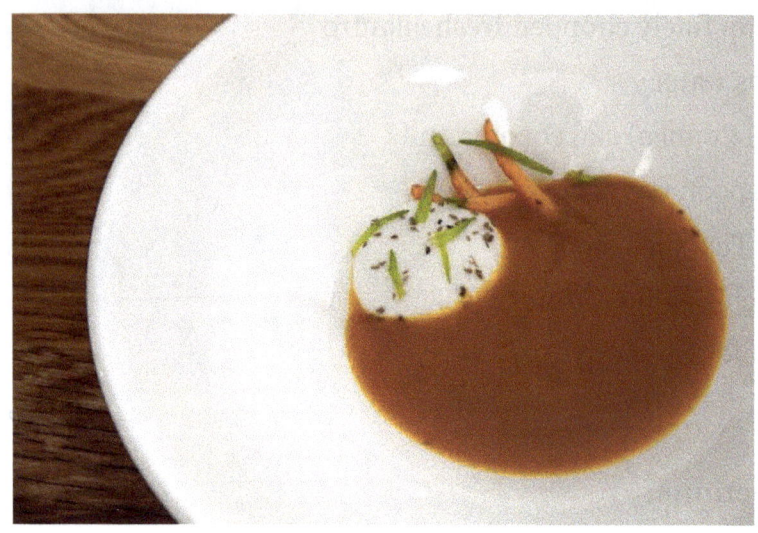

Ingredients

2 tablespoons extra virgin olive oil

1 small red onion, minced

1 medium carrot, peeled and thinly sliced

1 celery rib, thinly sliced

1/2 teaspoon dried tarragon

2 cups vegetable stock

1/4 cup wine vinegar

Directions:

Heat the oil over medium-high heat. Sauté red onions until tender for about 5 minutes. Slowly add carrots, celery, and tarragon Cook for another 5 minutes, or until carrots become tender. Add vegetable broth and vinegar Boil and simmer. Cook for 15 minutes longer.

Thai Carrot Soup

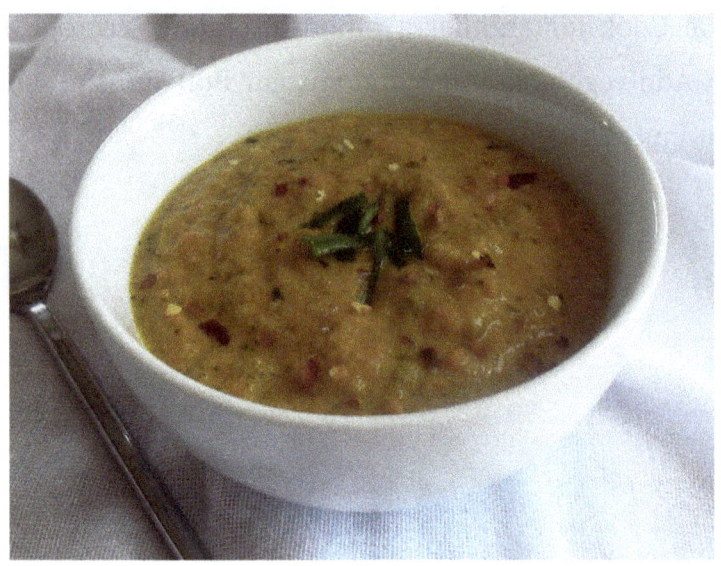

Ingredients

2 tablespoons sesame seed oil

1 small red onion, minced

1 small carrot, peeled and thinly sliced

1/2 teaspoon Thai chili paste

2 cups vegetable broth

1/4 cup coconut or white vinegar

1 sprig cilantro

Directions:

Heat the oil over medium-high heat. Sauté red onions until tender for about 5 minutes. Slowly add carrots and chili paste Cook for another 5 minutes, or until carrots become tender. Add vegetable stock and vinegar Boil and simmer. Cook for 15 minutes longer.

Hungarian Carrot Soup

Ingredients

2 tablespoons extra virgin olive oil

1 small red onion, minced

1 medium carrot, peeled and thinly sliced

1 celery rib, thinly sliced

5 garlic cloves finely minced

1 teaspoon Hungarian paprika

2 cups vegetable stock

1/4 cup wine vinegar

Directions:

Heat the oil over medium-high heat. Sauté red onions until tender for about 5 minutes. Slowly add carrots, celery, garlic cloves and Hungarian paprika Cook for another 5 minutes, or until carrots become tender. Add vegetable broth and vinegar Boil and simmer. Cook for 15 minutes longer.

French Red Soup

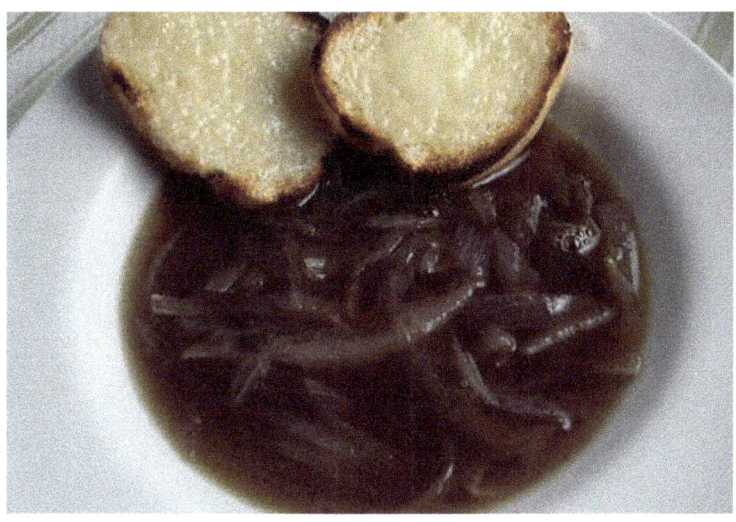

Ingredients

2 tablespoons olive oil

2 large red onions, minced

1 small turnip, peeled and thinly sliced

1 celery rib, thinly sliced

1/2 teaspoon herbs de Provence

1 cup vegetable stock

1 cup vegetable broth

1/4 cup wine vinegar

Directions:

Heat the oil over medium-high heat. Sauté red onions until tender for about 5 minutes. Slowly add turnip, celery, and herbs de Provence. Cook for another 5 minutes, or until turnip become tender. Add vegetable broth, stock and vinegar Boil and simmer. Cook for 15 minutes longer.

Vidalia Onion and Parsnip Soup

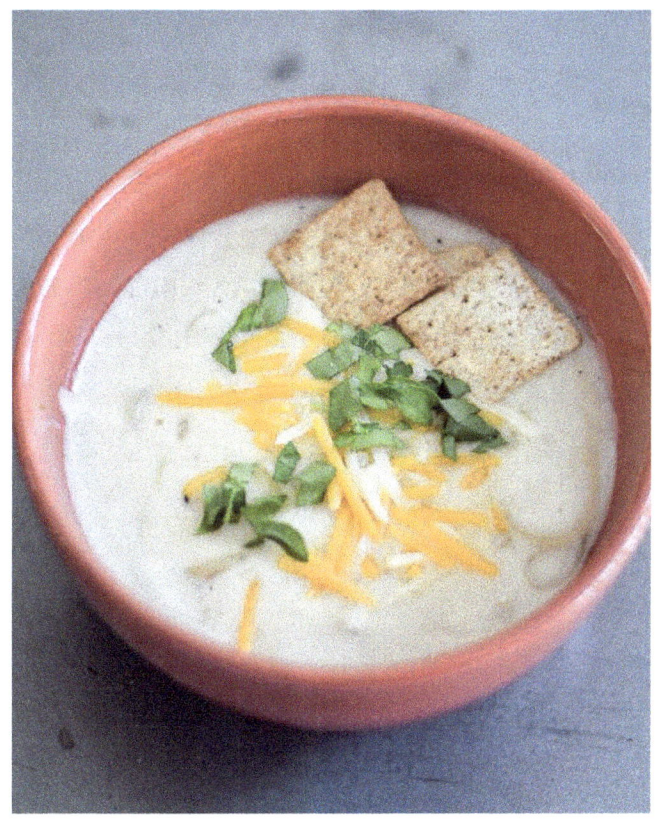

Ingredients

2 tablespoons extra virgin olive oil

3 Vidalia onions, minced

1 small parsnip, peeled and thinly sliced

1 celery rib, thinly sliced

1/2 teaspoon dried tarragon

2 cups vegetable stock

1/4 cup wine vinegar

Directions:

Heat the oil over medium-high heat. Sauté red onions until tender for about 5 minutes. Slowly add parsnip, celery, and tarragon Cook for another 5 minutes, or until carrots become tender. Add vegetable broth and vinegar Boil and simmer. Cook for 15 minutes longer.

Salad Tomato and Carrot Soup

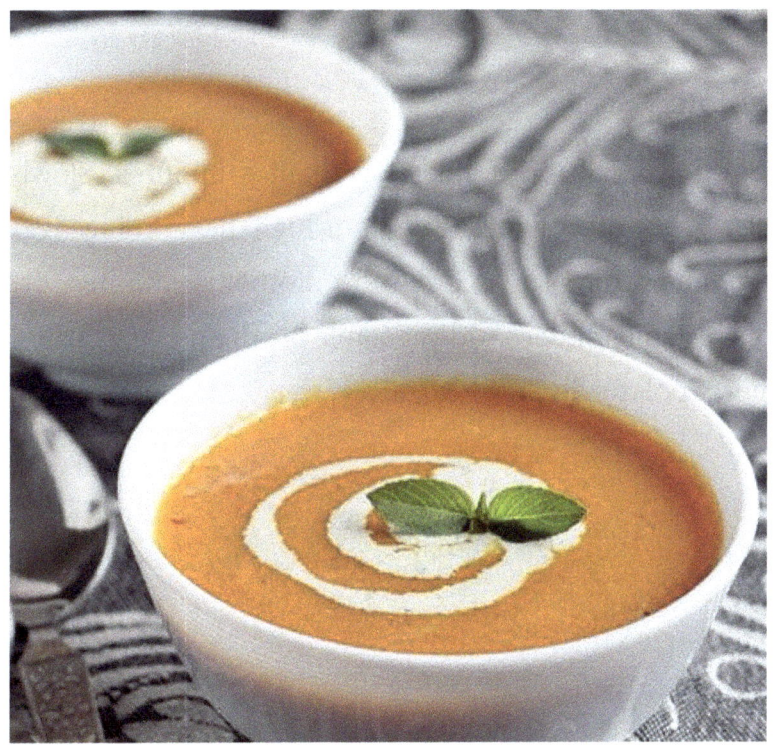

Ingredients

2 tablespoons olive oil

1 small red onion, minced

1 small carrot, peeled and thinly sliced

2 large Salad tomatoes, thinly sliced

1/2 teaspoon minced ginger

2 sprigs lemon grass

2 cups vegetable broth

2 tbsp. vinegar

Directions:

Sauté red onions until tender for about 5 minutes. Slowly add carrots, Heat the oil over medium-high heat. minced ginger, tomato, and lemon grass Cook for another 5 minutes, or until carrots become tender. Add vegetable broth and vinegar Boil and simmer. Cook for 15 minutes longer.

Baby Potato and Garbanzo Bean Soup

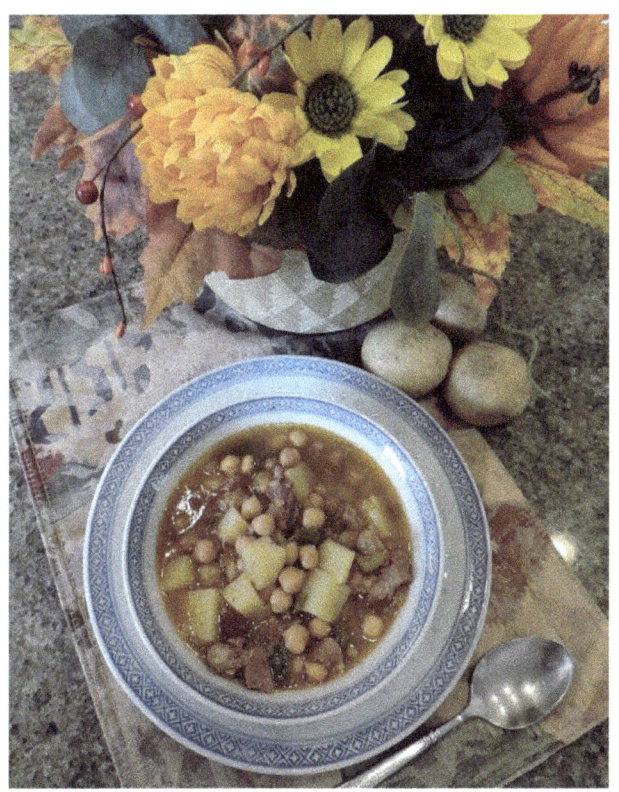

Ingredients

2 cups baby potatoes

3 tablespoons extra virgin olive oil, divided

2 ¼ cups cherry tomatoes

2 cups 1-inch cut fresh green beans

6 cloves garlic, minced

2 teaspoons dried basil

1 teaspoon flaked kosher salt

1 (15 ounce) can garbanzo beans drained and rinsed

2 teaspoons extra-virgin olive oil, or to taste (optional)

Sea salt Black pepper to taste

Directions:

Preheat your oven to 425 degrees F (220 degrees C). Line a baking pan with aluminum foil. Combine potatoes with 1 tablespoon olive oil in a medium bowl. Pour into the baking pan. Roast in the oven until tender, for about 30 minutes. Combine the cherry tomatoes, green beans, garlic, basil, and sea salt with 2 tablespoons of olive oil. Take potatoes out of the oven Push them to one side of the pan. Add the cherry tomato and green bean mixture. Roast until the tomatoes begin to wilt, for about 18 min. Take it out of the oven and pour into a dish. Add the garbanzo beans, 2 teaspoons olive oil, and season with salt and pepper.

French Baby Potato and Chick Pea Soup

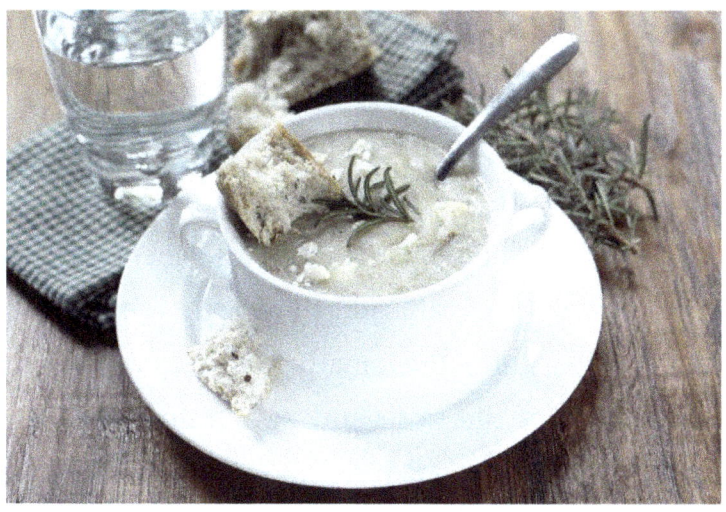

Ingredients

2 cups baby potatoes

3 tablespoons extra virgin olive oil, divided

2 ¼ cups Roma tomatoes

2 cups 1-inch cut fresh green beans

9 cloves garlic, minced

2 teaspoons herbs de Provence

1 teaspoon sea salt

1 (15 ounce) can chick peas, drained and rinsed

2 teaspoons extra-virgin olive oil, or to taste (optional)

Sea salt

Black pepper to taste

Directions:

Preheat your oven to 425 degrees F (220 degrees C). Line a baking pan with aluminum foil. Combine potatoes with 1 tablespoon olive oil in a medium bowl. Pour into the baking pan. Roast in the oven until tender, for about 30 minutes. Combine the cherry tomatoes, green beans, garlic, herbs de Provence, and sea salt with 2 tablespoons of olive oil. Take potatoes out of the oven Push them to one side of the pan. Add the cherry tomato and green bean mixture. Roast until the tomatoes begin to wilt, for about 18 min. Take it out of the oven and pour into a dish. Add the garbanzo beans, 2 teaspoons olive oil, and season with salt and pepper.

Soybean Soup

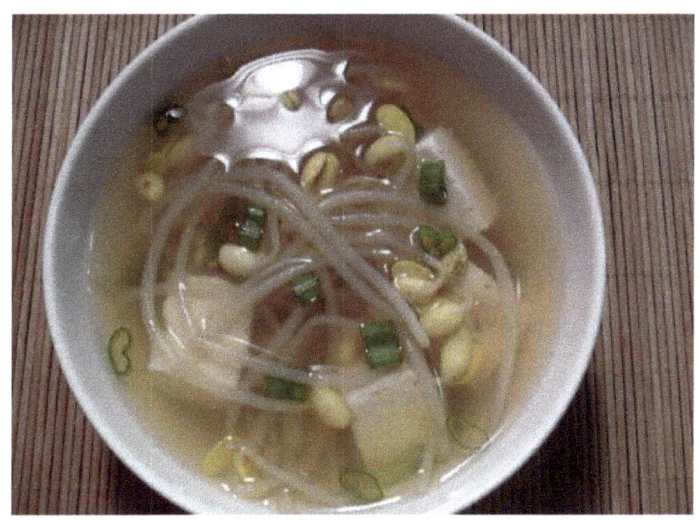

Ingredients

1 pound soy beans, sorted and rinsed

2 quarts veggie stock

1 medium onion, diced

5 cloves of garlic, peeled and smashed

2 tsp. sea salt

1/4 tsp white pepper

2 medium potatoes, diced

1 pound frozen, sliced carrots

3/4 cup chopped sun-dried tomatoes*

1-2 tsp dried dill

3-4 tbsp fresh, minced parsley

Directions:

Place the beans, stock, onion, garlic, sea salt and pepper in a pot Cook them over low-medium heat. Simmer for 3-4 hours, or longer, add water as needed. As the beans become soft, add the potato and simmer until potatoes become tender. Add the carrots, tomatoes and dill. Cook the carrots until heated thoroughly. Add the parsley, season with additional salt and white pepper.

Edamame Bean Soup

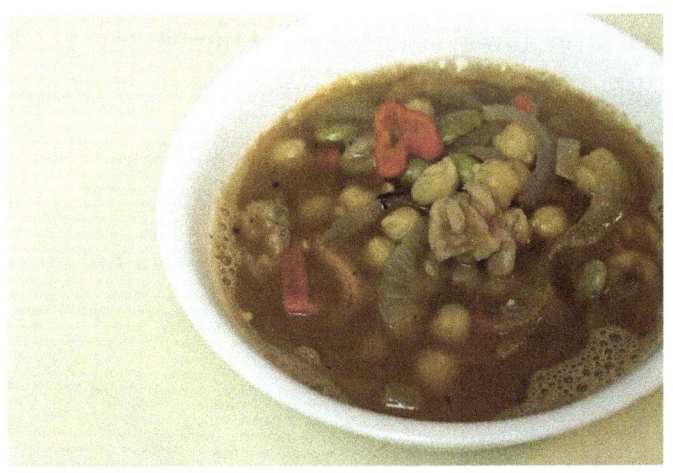

Ingredients

3/4 pound edamame beans, sorted and rinsed

2 quarts veggie broth

1 medium onion, diced

5 cloves of garlic, peeled and smashed

2 tsp. sea salt

1/4 tsp black pepper

2 medium potatoes, diced

1 pound frozen, sliced carrots

3/4 cup chopped sun-dried tomatoes*

1-2 tsp dried dill

3-4 tbsp fresh, minced parsley

Directions:

Place the beans, broth, onion, garlic, sea salt and pepper in a pot Cook them over low-medium heat. Simmer for 3-4 hours, or longer, add water as needed. As the beans become soft, add the potato and simmer until potatoes become tender. Add the carrots, tomatoes and dill. Cook the carrots until heated thoroughly. Add the parsley, season with additional salt and black pepper.

Peas and Kidney Bean Soup with Parsnips

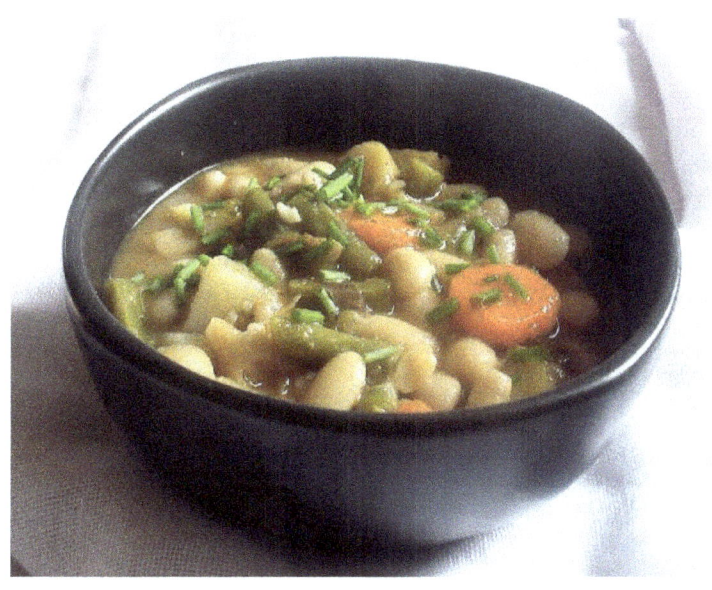

Ingredients

1/2 pound dried peas, sorted and rinsed

¼ pound dried kidney beans, sorted and rinsed

¼ pound garbanzo beans, sorted and rinsed

2 quarts veggie stock

2 medium red onion, diced

5 cloves of garlic, peeled and smashed

2 tsp. sea salt

1/4 tsp black pepper

2 medium potatoes, diced

1 pound frozen, sliced parsnips

3/4 cup chopped sun-dried tomatoes*

1-2 tsp dried dill

3-4 tbsp fresh, minced parsley

Directions:

Place the beans, stock, onion, garlic, sea salt and pepper in a pot Cook them over low-medium heat. Simmer for 3-4 hours, or longer, add water as needed. As the beans become soft, add the potato and simmer until potatoes become tender. Add the carrots, tomatoes and dill. Cook the carrots until heated thoroughly. Add the parsley, season with additional salt and black pepper.

Winter Squash and Turnip Soup

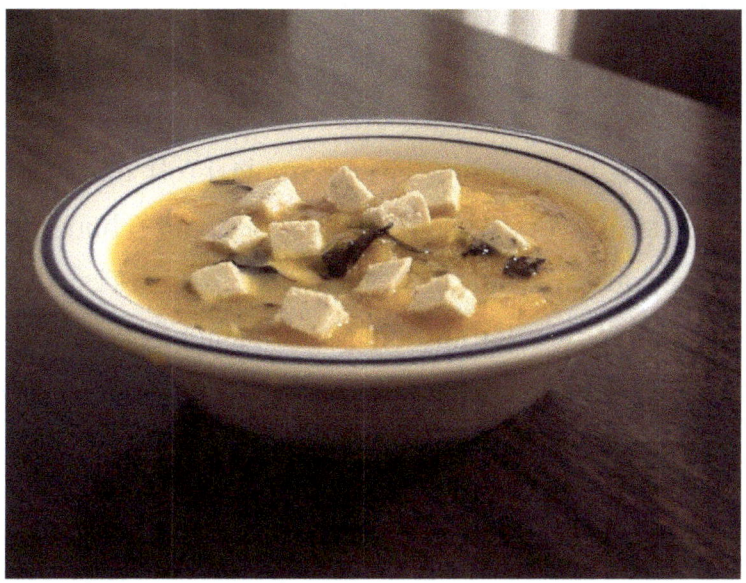

Ingredients

1 medium winter squash (1 lb of peeled and cubed butternut squash)

1 medium red onion, diced

2/3 lb, peeled and cut into chunks

1 turnip, peeled and sliced

3 cups vegetable broth

1 bay leaf

1 tsp sea salt

1 tsp white pepper

1/4 tsp dried ground sage

½ can coconut milk

Directions:

Combine the squash, onion, carrots, apple, broth and bay leaf in a slow cooker. Cover and cook on low for about 6 hours or until veggies are soft. Take out the bay leaf and discard. Transfer these Ingredients to a blender and blend until smooth Pour it back to the slow cooker Season with salt, pepper & sage Pour the coconut milk. Add more salt and pepper to taste.

Winter Squash and Carrot Soup

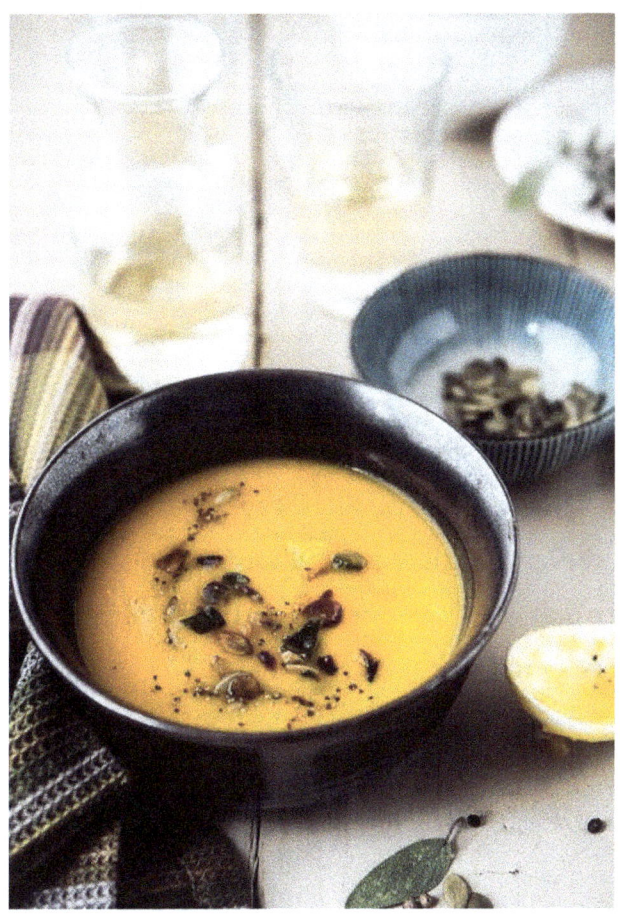

Ingredients

1 medium winter squash

1 medium yellow onion, diced

2/3 lb carrots, peeled and cut into chunks

1 Fuji apple, peeled and sliced

3 cups vegetable broth

1 Italian seasoning

1 tsp sea salt

1 tsp white pepper

1/4 tsp dried ground sage

½ can almond milk

Directions:

Combine the squash, onion, carrots, apple, broth and Italian seasoning in a slow cooker. Cover and cook on low for about 6 hours or until veggies are soft. Transfer these Ingredients to a blender and blend until smooth Pour it back to the slow cooker Season with salt, pepper & sage Pour the almond milk. Add more salt and pepper to taste.

Hubbard Squash and Parsnip Soup

Ingredients

1lb. hubbard squash, cubed

1 medium yellow onion, diced

2/3 lb parsnips, peeled and cut into chunks

1 pear peeled and sliced

3 cups vegetable broth

1 cilantro

1 tsp sea salt

1 tsp white pepper

½ can almond milk

Directions:

Combine the squash, yellow onion, parsnips, pears, broth and cilantro in a slow cooker. Cover and cook on low for about 6 hours or until veggies are soft. Transfer these Ingredients to a blender and blend until smooth Pour it back to the slow cooker Season with salt & pepper Pour the almond milk. Add more salt and pepper to taste.

Curried Winter Squash Curry

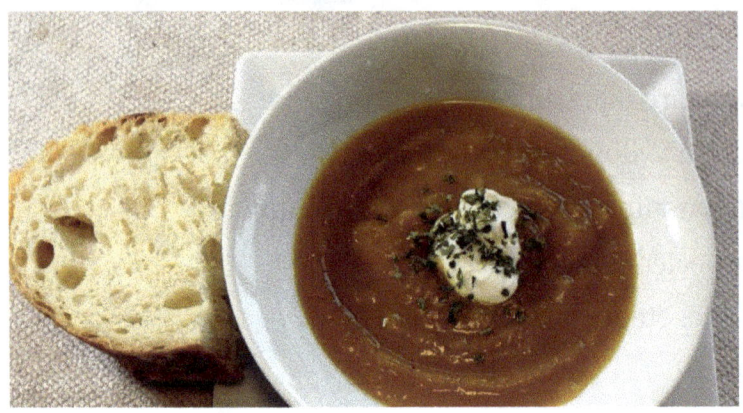

Ingredients

1 medium winter squash (1 lb of peeled and cubed butternut squash)

1 medium red onion, diced

2/3 lb parsnips, peeled and cut into chunks

1 Fuji apple, peeled and sliced

3 cups vegetable broth

1 tsp. curry powder

3 Thai bird chilies, finely chopped

1 tsp sea salt

1 tsp white pepper

1/4 tsp Thai basil

½ can coconut milk

Directions:

Combine the squash, onion, parsnips, apple, broth, Thai bird chilies and curry powder a slow cooker. Cover and cook on low for about 6 hours or until veggies are soft. Take out the bay leaf and discard. Transfer these Ingredients to a blender and blend until smooth Pour it back to the slow cooker Season with salt, pepper & Thai basil Pour the coconut milk. Add more salt and pepper to taste.

Garbanzo Bean Tortilla and Taco Soup

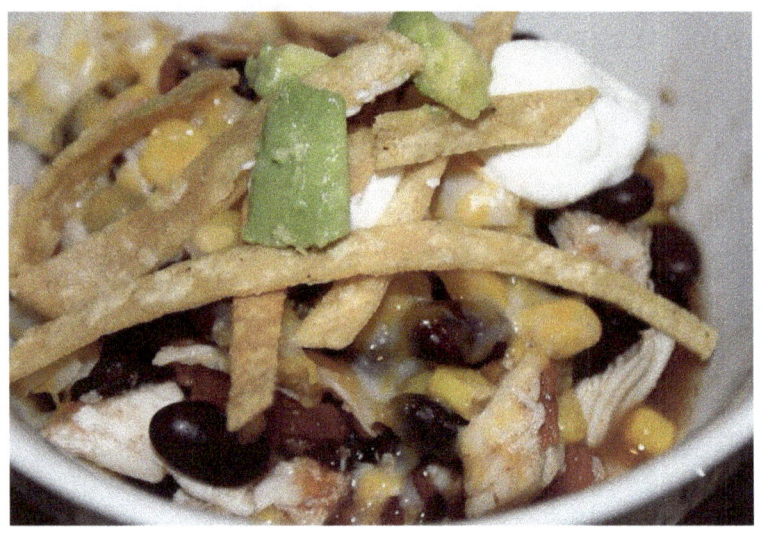

Ingredients:

1 teaspoon extra-virgin olive oil

1/2 cup chopped onions

4 cloves garlic, minced

1 cup vegetable broth

1 cup vegetable stock

1 cup salsa

1 14-ounce can garbanzo beans

1 green bell pepper, chopped

1/2 teaspoon salt

1 avocado, chopped

1/2 cup loosely-packed cilantro

Directions:

Add onions and garlic to saucepan and sauté until softened. Add the stock, salsa, bell peppers, beans, and salt. Bring to a boil over high heat. Reduce to low and simmer for 5 minutes. Garnish with half of the avocado, cilantro, and tortilla chips.

Lentils and Annatto Seed Tortilla Soup

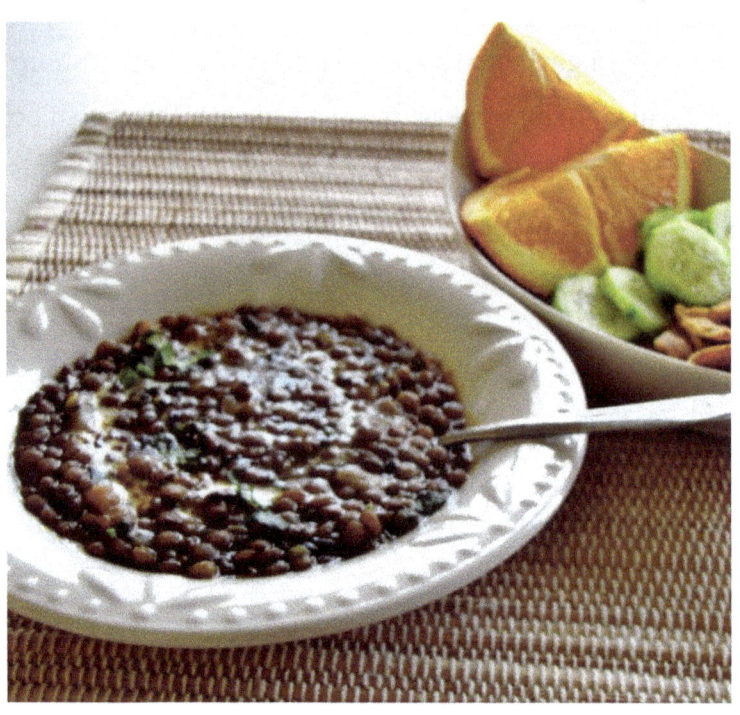

Ingredients:

1 teaspoon extra-virgin olive oil

1/2 cup chopped onions

4 cloves garlic, minced

1 tsp. annatto seeds

1 orange, peeled

1 cup vegetable broth

1 cup vegetable stock

1 cup salsa

1 14-ounce can lentils

1 green bell pepper, chopped

1/2 teaspoon salt

1 avocado, chopped

1/2 cup loosely-packed cilantro

Optional:

1/2 cup crumbled corn tortilla chips

Add olive oil to a pan and heat it to medium.

Directions:

Add onions and garlic to saucepan and sauté until softened. Add the stock, salsa, bell peppers, beans, orange, annatto seeds and salt. Bring to a boil over high heat. Reduce to low and simmer for 5 minutes. Garnish with half of the avocado, cilantro, and tortilla chips. Remove the orange

Habanero Mung Bean Taco Soup

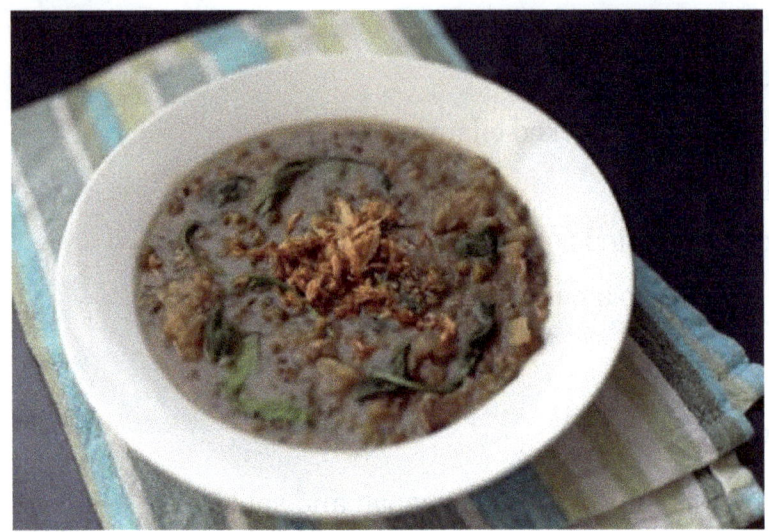

Ingredients:

1 teaspoon extra-virgin olive oil

1/2 cup chopped onions

4 cloves garlic, minced

1 cup vegetable broth

1 cup vegetable stock

1 cup salsa

1 14-ounce can mung beans

1/4 habanero chili, chopped

1/2 teaspoon salt

1 tsp. annatto seed powder

1 avocado, chopped

1/2 cup loosely-packed cilantro

Directions:

Add onions and garlic to saucepan and sauté until softened. Add the stock, salsa, habanero pepper, beans, annatto seed powder and salt. Bring to a boil over high heat. Reduce to low and simmer for 5 minutes. Garnish with half of the avocado, cilantro, and tortilla chips.

Borlotti Bean and Pepper Soup

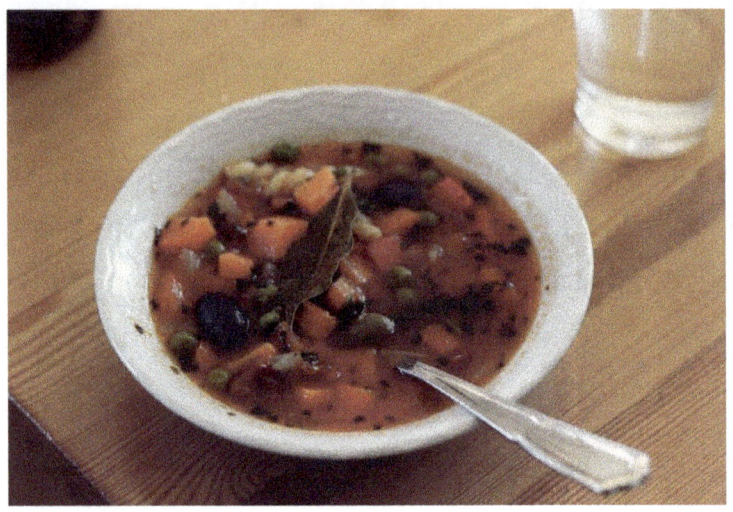

Ingredients:

1 teaspoon extra-virgin olive oil

1/2 cup chopped onions

4 cloves garlic, minced

1 ½ cup vegetable broth

½ cup vegetable stock

1 cup salsa

1 14-ounce can borlotti beans

1 red bell pepper, chopped

1 green red bell pepper

½ tsp. all spice

¼ tsp. oregano

1/2 teaspoon salt

1 avocado, chopped

1/2 cup loosely-packed cilantro

Directions:

Optional:

1/2 cup crumbled corn tortilla chips Add olive oil to a pan and heat it to medium. Add onions and garlic to saucepan and sauté until softened. Add the stock, salsa, red and green bell peppers, beans, all spice, oregano, and salt. Bring to a boil over high heat. Reduce to low and simmer for 5 minutes. Garnish with half of the avocado, cilantro, and tortilla chips.

Turnip and Chili Soup

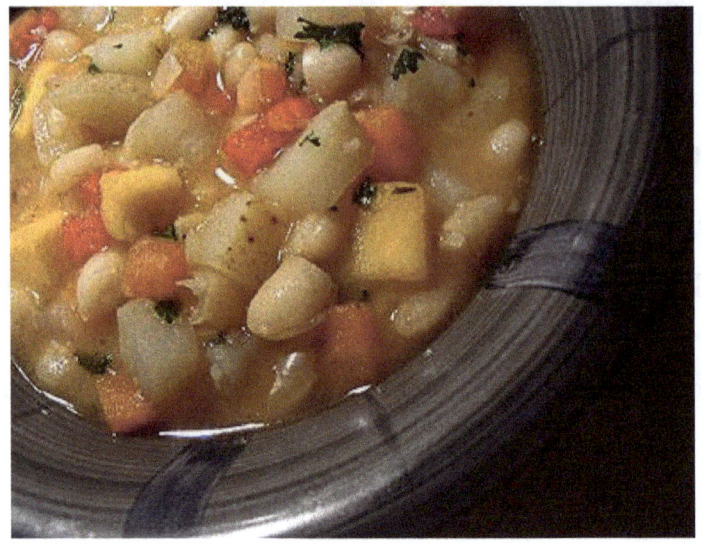

Ingredients

1 tablespoon extra virgin olive oil

2 teaspoon crushed garlic

1 tablespoon chopped fresh cilantro

1 teaspoon chili paste

1 red onion, chopped

3 large turnips, peeled and sliced

Sea salt to taste

1 large potato, peeled and chopped

5 cups vegetable broth

Directions:

Heat oil over medium heat. Cook the garlic, cilantro and chili paste. Stir fry the onion until tender. Add the turnips and potato. Cook for 5 minutes and add the vegetable broth. Simmer until potatoes and turnips are soft. Blend until smooth.

Spicy Squash Soup

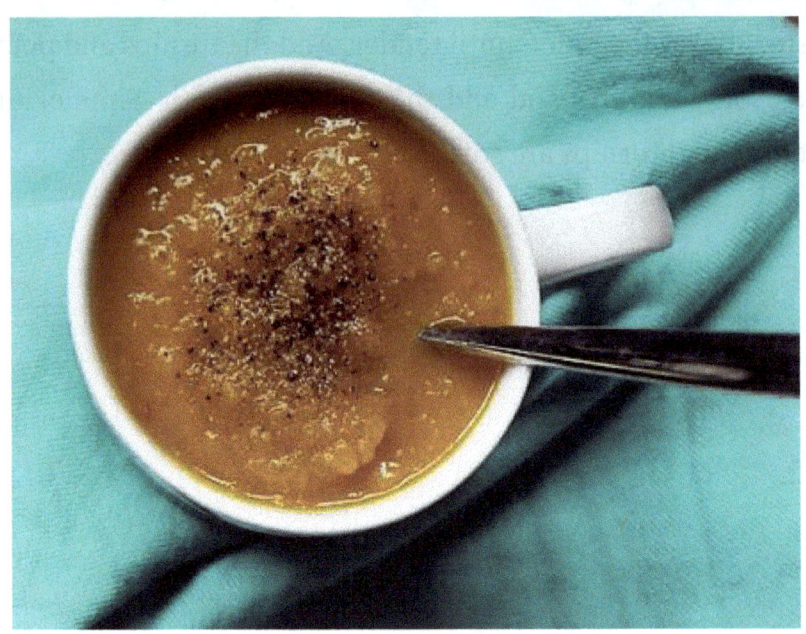

Ingredients

1 tablespoon canola oil

2 teaspoon crushed garlic

1 tablespoon chopped fresh cilantro

1 teaspoon Sriracha sauce

1 tbsp. rice wine vinegar

1 red onion, chopped

3 pcs. of small summer squash, peeled and sliced

Sea salt to taste

½ cup shitake mushrooms, stemmed and coarsely chopped

5 cups vegetable broth

Directions:

Heat oil over medium heat. Cook the garlic, cilantro, rice wine vinegar, mushrooms and Sriracha hot sauce. Stir fry the onion until tender. Add the summer squash and potato. Cook for 5 minutes and add the vegetable broth. Simmer until potatoes and squash are soft. Blend until smooth.

Jalapeno Butternut Squash Soup

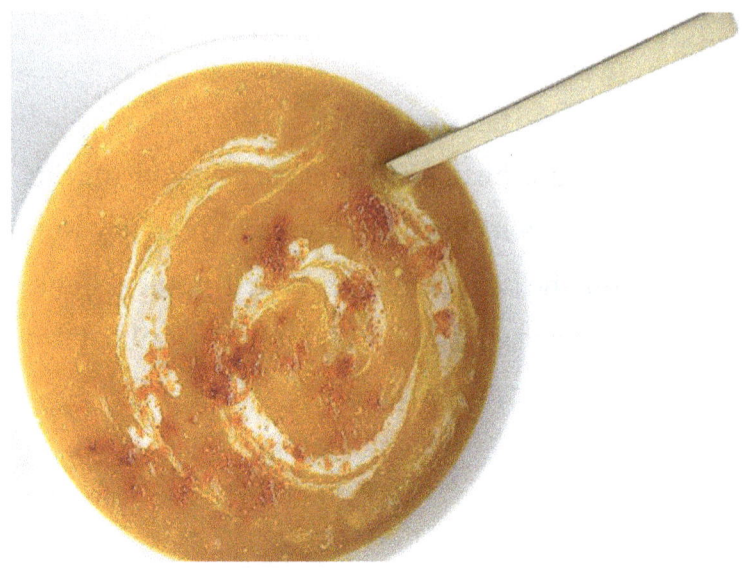

Ingredients

1 tablespoon extra virgin olive oil

2 teaspoon crushed garlic

1 tablespoon chopped fresh cilantro

1 teaspoon chili paste

1 teaspoon limejuice

1 teaspoon jalapeno, coarsely chopped

1 red onion, chopped

3 pcs. butternut squash, peeled and sliced

Sea salt to taste

1 large potato, peeled and chopped

5 cups vegetable broth

Directions:

Heat oil over medium heat. Cook the garlic, cilantro, lime, cumin, jalapeno and chili paste. Stir fry the onion until tender. Add the butternut squash and potato. Cook for 5 minutes and add the vegetable broth. Simmer until potatoes and squash are soft. Blend until smooth.

Miso Summer Squash and Sweet Potato Soup

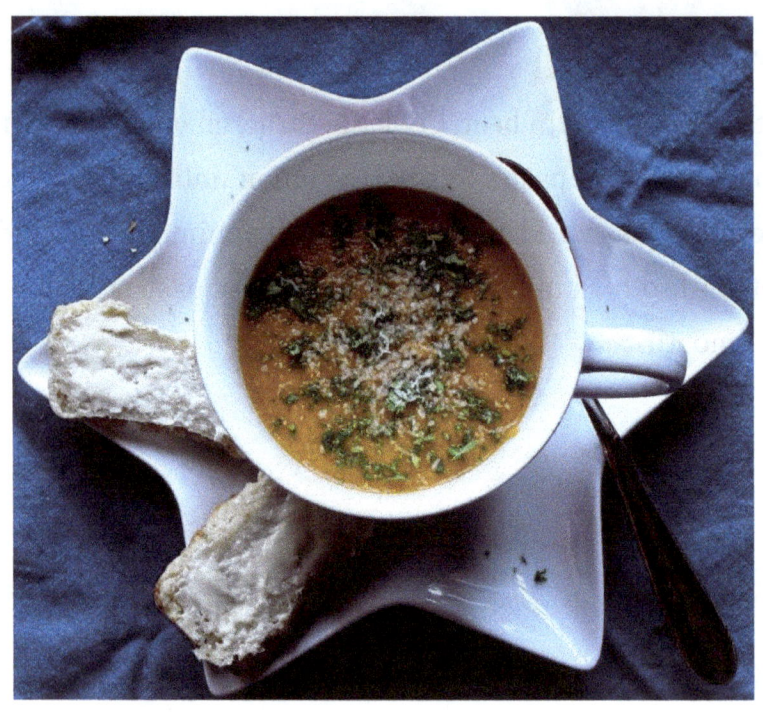

Ingredients

1 tablespoon non-dairy butter oil

4 teaspoon crushed garlic

1 red onion, chopped

5 tsp. miso paste

3 large summer squash, peeled and sliced

Sea salt to taste

1 large sweet potato, peeled and chopped

3 cups vegetable broth

2 cups almond milk

Directions:

Heat non-dairy butter over medium heat. Cook the garlic, cilantro and chili paste. Stir fry the onion until tender. Add the summer squash and potato. Cook for 5 minutes and add the almond milk, miso paste and vegetable broth. Simmer until potatoes and summer squash are soft. Blend until smooth.

Middle Eastern Inspired Creamy Squash Soup

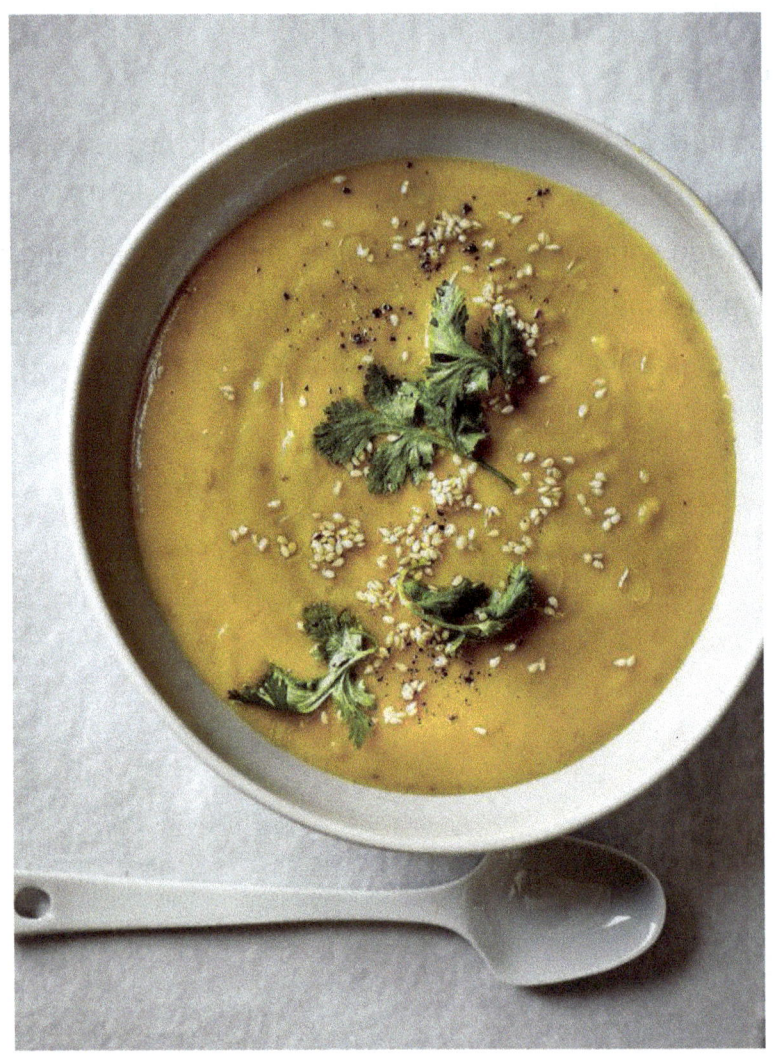

Ingredients

4 tablespoons extra virgin olive oil

1 small red onion, coarsely chopped

1 large leek, white part only, sliced

1 green bell pepper, coarsely chopped

2 pcs. small dry-roasted poblano chili, sliced

8 cloves garlic, diced

½ tsp. turmeric

¾ tsp. cumin

1 tbsp. dried parsley

1 tbsp lemon juice

1 large squash, cubed (you can use two if you like your soup thick)

4 cups vegetable broth

1 cup cashews

1-1/4 cup almond milk

Sea Salt

Black pepper, to taste

Directions:

Optional garnish: Sliced jalapeno pepper Soak the cashews in almond milk for half an hour. Heat the olive oil in a pan. Cook the onion, leek, chilies, green bell pepper, garlic, and squash over low heat until the onion is translucent. Add the broth, turmeric, cumin, parsley and lemon juice into the pan. Simmer until the squash are fork tender, about 25 min. Remove from the heat. Pour into a blender and blend until smooth. Clean the blender. Blend cashews with the milk until smooth Stir this into the soup. Heat on medium for a few minutes. Garnish with slices of jalapeno chili.

Habanero and Ancho Chili Sweet Potato Soup

Ingredients

4 tablespoons organic butter

1 small red onion, coarsely chopped

1 large leek, white part only, sliced

1 ancho chili, coarsely chopped

1 (or two if you like things spicy) small dry-roasted poblano chili, sliced

9 cloves garlic, diced

1 large sweet potato, cubed (you can use two if you like your soup thick)

4 cups vegetable broth

1 cup kidney beans

1-1/4 cup almond milk

½ tsp. cumin

1 habanero pepper, coarsely chopped

Sea Salt

Black pepper, to taste

Directions:

Optional garnish: Sliced jalapeno pepper Soak the cashews in almond milk for half an hour. Melt non-dairy butter in a pan.

Cook the onion, leek, chilies, garlic, and potato over low heat until the onion is translucent. Add the broth, cumin and habanero pepper into the pan. Simmer until the potatoes are fork tender, about 25 min. Remove from the heat. Pour into a blender and blend until smooth. Clean the blender. Blend cashews with the milk until smooth Stir this into the soup. Heat on medium for a few minutes. Garnish with slices of jalapeno chili.

www.ingramcontent.com/pod-product-compliance
Lightning Source LLC
Chambersburg PA
CBHW071113030426
42336CB00013BA/2062